Dennen's FORCEPS DELIVERIES

Fourth Edition

Edited by Ralph W. Hale, MD, FACOG

Executive Vice President
The American College of
Obstetricians and Gynecologists
Washington, DC

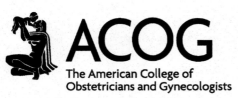

ACOG
The American College of
Obstetricians and Gynecologists

409 12th Street SW
Washington, DC 20024-2188

Illustrations: The drawings were done by Mr. Alfred Fineberg, Medical Artist, Columbia University, New York

Note: These guidelines should not be construed as dictating an exclusive course of treatment or procedure. Variations in practice may be warranted based on the needs of the individual patient, resources, and limitations unique to the institution or type of practice.

Library of Congress Cataloging-in-Publication Data

Dennen's forceps deliveries.— 4th ed./edited by Ralph W. Hale
    p.; cm.
  Includes bibliographical references and index.
  ISBN: 978-0-915473-70-0 (hardcover)
       978-1-948258-40-1 (paperback)
       978-1-948258-06-7 (ebook)
  1. Delivery (Obstetrics) 2. Obstetrical forceps. I. Title: Forceps
    deliveries. II. Hale, Ralph W., 1935- III. Dennen, Edward Henry,
    1896- Forceps deliveries.
    [DNLM: 1. Delivery—methods. 2. Obstetrical Forceps. WQ 425
    D398f2001]
  RG739 .D4 2001
  618.8'2—dc21

                                  2001022346

Printed in the United States of America

2345/5432

Contents

Foreword to the Third Edition

*F*or many reasons, some good, some very bad, the forceps operation has come close to extinction in this country over the past decade or two. This, in my opinion, is a highly undesirable development, and I was delighted to hear that the author and the publishers of this book are reacting to a virtual demand from obstetricians that the older edition be updated. Happily, there is an increasing realization among obstetricians that the near abandonment of the forceps operation in recent years has not been advantageous to gravida or their fetuses.

The generation of obstetricians that I represent was trained to use forceps with great frequency, even routinely. We believed that the advantages of the obstetric forceps far outweighed the disadvantages and that their use could move us closer to our stated goals of a healthy mother and a well child. In my opinion, that idea remains sound, although experience has demanded that we balance the risks and advantages of forceps against the well-known shortcomings of abdominal surgery. Cesarean delivery is much safer than it was 30–40 years ago but still carries a maternal risk of death that is several times greater than that for vaginal delivery. This fact is often forgotten today in favor of fetal health and survival. However, both the mother and the fetus-neonate must be considered in obstetric decisions. In the face of higher maternal mortality from abdominal delivery, it seems reasonable to consider a forceps delivery as an alternative when a cesarean delivery is to be performed for "failure to progress." Much of the time, the use of forceps will be rejected outright (because, eg, the pelvis is too small or the station of the vertex is too high), but in a certain proportion of cases (the exact frequency being dependent on the skill of the operator as well as other factors), the forceps operation still appears to be desirable and preferable.

There is a serious need for a book that illustrates in an encyclopedic way the intricacies of obstetric forceps usage. The present volume is an admirable fulfillment of that need. It was written originally by an acknowledged authority on forceps delivery and was updated by his talented son, who, coincidentally, was a medical-school friend of mine. The descriptions of forceps techniques in the older edition could not be improved upon and are included intact from the earlier edition. The present author has updated the indications and contraindications of the forceps operation and has put in perspective the usefulness of forceps in an obstetric milieu quite unlike that of the prior generation. The result of their joint work is that Dennen's *Forceps Deliveries* is authoritative, readable, and certain to become a new classic on a reemerging and important area of obstetrics.

Kenneth R. Niswander, MD, FACOG
Professor Obstetrics and Gynecology
University of California at Davis

Note: The editor has maintained this foreword in the fourth edition because it succinctly describes the situation at the time the third edition was published in 1989. For the obstetrician, the passing of forceps as an integral part of the practice of obstetrics should not result in a loss of a significant component of the history of obstetrics.

Preface

*F*or many obstetricians trained in the 1930s through the 1960s, the use of forceps was an integral and important part of day-to-day practice. The variety of types of forceps and their indications were a critical part of the education of an obstetrician. This book was first published in 1947 by Dr. Edward Dennen to be used as a guide in this educational process. Other editions followed in 1955, 1965, and 1989. The last edition was edited by Dr. Philip Dennen, son of Dr. Edward Dennen. Since the time that the earlier editions were published and that I, like many of my contemporaries, learned the art and skill of forceps delivery, the care of the obstetric patient has evolved. No longer are forceps in common use in the labor and delivery areas of hospitals. Cesarean delivery now occurs at a rate of 20–25% and has replaced the use of forceps in many situations.

Nevertheless, the use of forceps and an understanding of that use still are critical components of obstetric practice. When the American College of Obstetricians and Gynecologists (ACOG) learned that the publisher of this book had determined that there was insufficient demand to justify a revision or republishing of this text, an offer was made to buy the rights for the book. This edition is a result of the successful completion of that effort and of the College's commitment to supply a time-proven resource for the use of forceps.

This edition has been significantly revised to reflect the current status of forceps deliveries and to incorporate the changes taking place as we enter a new century. Previous discussions of special types of forceps have been relegated to the section on history, and a new chapter has been added on vacuum assisted delivery, which includes evidence-based recommendations regarding its use. Wherever possible, the original language and explanations by the original author have been maintained to preserve the classic nature of the book.

This new edition was made available through ACOG's Development Committee, whose funds are provided by College members to assist in projects outside regular College activities. As such, it can be truthfully stated that the effort to continue the availability of Dr. Dennen's book, *Forceps Deliveries*, is one made on the part of obstetrician–gynecologists.

Ralph W. Hale, MD, FACOG
ACOG Executive Vice President

Preface to the Third Edition

orceps Deliveries had its origin in the *Manual of Forceps Deliveries*, privately published by Dr. Edward H. Dennen in 1947. The Manual was used by his residents and his students at the Cornell Medical College and the New York Polyclinic Postgraduate Medical School. The book, completed with illustrations, evolved and was published by F.A. Davis in 1955. A second edition of *Forceps Deliveries* followed in 1965. It has now been out of print for many years. Numerous requests for copies have been received from practicing physicians, residents, and program directors. I have been told that a few copies that did not disappear from hospital libraries are protected and (as in my hospital) copied by individuals for their use.

Although the obstetric goals of a healthy mother and infant are unchanged since 1965, the means to that end have become radically altered. The day of the 4% cesarean delivery rate is long gone, but so also is the day of the 50 per 1,000 neonatal mortality rate. Technology, medicine in general, and society in particular have induced changes in obstetric thinking and practice. Too frequently, operators with forceps ability are made aware, following a successful delivery, that in other institutions or in other hands a damaged infant could only have been avoided by abdominal delivery. This is the reason for this book.

Many parts of the book are virtually unchanged from the original version, and credit belongs to the senior Dr. Dennen. In particular, descriptions of technique have stood the tests of time and also the specific efforts of an inquisitive son who, in over 30 years of active clinical practice and teaching, was unable to find a better way to perform or describe them. Material considered obsolescent or in conflict with modern obstetrics has been deleted. The 1988 American College of Obstetricians and Gynecologists forceps classification is used as reference. Alterations and additions to the book reflect current obstetric literature and are an effort to make Forceps Deliveries pertinent and useful to both student and clinician.

Philip C. Dennen, MD, FACOG

Note: This preface appeared in the third edition. Because it gives a unique insight into the original author and subsequent author, the Editor believes it should be included in this edition as well.

Dennen's Forceps Deliveries

Fourth Edition

CHAPTER 1

Historic Review

*T*he history of the obstetric forceps is long and often colorful. Evidence of single or paired instruments in Sanskrit writings dates from about 1500 bc. Egyptian, Greek, Roman, and Arabic writings picture or refer to forceps, although it is presumed that most of these instruments were used for the extraction of a dead fetus. Credit for the invention of the precursor of the modern instruments for use on live infants goes to Peter Chamberlin (ca. 1600) of England. Gene Palfyn (1649–1730) of Ghent independently invented a paired "mains de fer." William Smellie, in 1745, described the accurate application of forceps and rotation of the fetus to occiput anterior presentation, rather than the previously practiced pelvic application with traction regardless of the position of the head. The addition of a pelvic curve to the forceps is ascribed to Smellie and independently to André Levret (1747), who also developed the French lock. Etienne Tarnier (1877) initiated the concept of axis traction with a new instrument. Inventions, modifications, reinventions, and variants have led to the description of over 700 obstetric forceps. Most of these, although fascinating, are of greatest significance only to the obstetric historian.

For centuries, the concept of forceps was of an extricating tool, usually used in desperation as a last resort in a difficult situation. Prior to the advent of antibiotics, intravenous fluids, blood transfusion, and safe anesthesia, abdominal delivery carried horrendous maternal risk. Vaginal delivery was thus mandatory, contributing to the reputation of forceps as being associated with trauma and often tragedy.

In 1845, Sir James Simpson designed a forceps that was scientifically calculated to the appropriate cephalic and pelvic curvatures. He encouraged the use of the forceps because "the infantile mortality attended upon parturition increases in a ratio progressive with the increased duration of labor." Joseph DeLee modified that instrument and in 1920 presented his concept of the prophylactic forceps operation, asserting that the procedure protected both the maternal tissues and the fetal brain. This theory has never been scientifically proven or disproven. Although Dr. DeLee was criticized by his colleagues for interfering with nature, the concept of elective forceps was increasingly popular with practicing obstetricians. Many authors in the 1930s and 1940s reported superior outcomes for the fetus with the use of low forceps and episiotomy as compared with spontaneous delivery. Many institutions reported forceps use in over 50% of deliveries.

Forceps designers, and their satellites and students who became teachers, taught the use only of their favorite instruments. Other types were ignored except to emphasize their disadvantages. The numerous types once in general use indicate that there is no universal forceps. Many an operator experienced a sense of relief and the thrill of success after the use of one type of forceps after failure of another type on the same patient. The reasons why one pair of forceps succeeded after another had failed came to represent the advantages of the former and the disadvantages of the latter.

Factors were at work to slow, then reverse, the swing of the pendulum as cesarean delivery techniques improved. The safety of cesarean birth, along with the availability of blood replacement and antibiotics, made it a better alternative than a difficult forceps delivery. Other forceps indications were removed by the increased use of oxytocin in the treatment of dysfunctional labor and by improved methods of monitoring fetal status. Decreased use of general anesthesia with increased and improved conduction anesthesia techniques, though adding a few cases in which forceps were preferred, subtracted more. By the 1980s, the use of forceps had declined significantly.

The status of forceps in modern obstetrics is constantly under discussion within the specialty. Controversy is only proper in the effort for improvement of results. As a result, many forceps types are now used sparingly while others have been dropped from use completely.

The advent of special types of forceps was accompanied by advantages as well as disadvantages and required different techniques of application and traction. A thorough knowledge of the advantages and disadvantages of the various types of forceps, as well as the techniques for their use, was required in order to eliminate many of the adverse outcomes that resulted from following blind faith in one type or from using the "trial-and-error" method.

Because today's resident will only rarely be exposed to several of these forceps types, they are mentioned here for historic reasons.

Barton Forceps

Dr. Lyman G. Barton of Plattsburg, New York, designed his forceps for application to heads arrested in the transverse diameter of the inlet, especially those with a posterior parietal presentation. The instrument may be used to advantage in deep transverse arrest, oblique posterior position, and, rarely, in face presentation. The Barton forceps was presented in 1925 (Figure 1–1).

One blade is attached to the shank by a hinge, making it flexible over an arc of 90 degrees. The other blade has a deep cephalic curve. The blades are solid and are attached to the shanks laterally at an angle of about 50 degrees, so that when the forceps is held in the anterior position, there is no pelvic curve. However, when it is rotated over an arc of 90 degrees to the transverse position, the angle of attachment of the blades to the shanks forms a perfect pelvic curve. The lock is of the sliding type. There is a separate traction handle that can be applied to give axis traction. The use of the traction handle is advised because it greatly facilitates the mechanics of use of the instrument. It also aids the operator to think in terms of the long axis of the head. This is important in light of the difference between the Barton forceps and classical instruments.

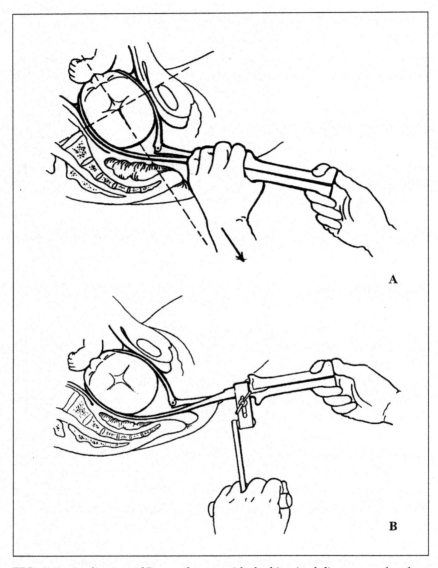

FIG. 1–1. Application of Barton forceps with the biparietal diameter at the plane of the inlet. The transverse arrest as pictured would be a high forceps. The technique is no different at mid or low forceps levels. **A.** Application of Barton forceps in left occiput transverse presentation. Any asynclitism has been corrected by equalizing the handles. **B.** Barton forceps with axis-traction handle, ready for traction in left occiput transverse presentation. Anterior rotation is not performed until the head is near the outlet.

The thin, hinged blade of the Barton forceps affords an easy and accurate application, via the "wandering" maneuver, to transverse heads, particularly those in posterior parietal presentation. The hinge allows the blade to be wandered around the head into place in front of the anterior ear, behind the symphysis. The sliding lock allows for correction of asynclitism, as locking can be accomplished at any level on the shank. The traction handle provides good axis traction. The most important indication for the use of this instrument was in a flat pelvis with a head arrested at mid-pelvis in the transverse diameter.

Hawks–Dennen Forceps

A light, fixed axis traction forceps, best suited to any anterior position of the head, was designed by E. M. Hawks and E. H. Dennen. The blades are a modification of the Simpson type (see Chapter 2, "Classical Instruments"). The long cephalic curve of the Hawks–Dennen forceps has lengthened tips and an exaggerated curve of the posterior lips. The fenestrated blades have beveled inner surfaces, decreasing the risk of bruising or cutting. The shanks are a modification of the Piper instrument, having a reverse pelvic curve in the middle, although shorter and with a sharper curve than that of the Piper. The curve in the shanks is such that the finger guards lie in the long axis of the head when the forceps are properly applied. This results in axis traction in all cases (Figures 1–2 and 1–3).

The Hawks–Dennen instrument may be used as a primary tractor or after rotation by another instrument when a better traction device is desired. The longer cephalic curve fits molded heads evenly, and the toes seat well below the malar eminences. In positions other than occiput in an anterior quadrant, however, other instruments are preferable. Exceptions to this caveat would be in the case of delivery as an occiput posterior, mentum anterior, or aftercoming head.

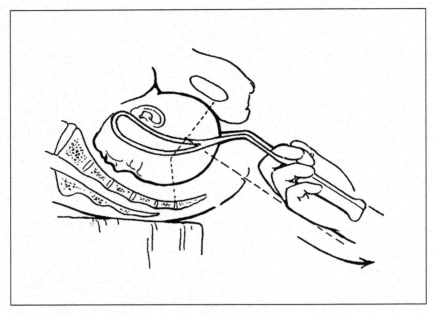

FIG. 1–2. Instrumental axis traction with Hawks–Dennen forceps.

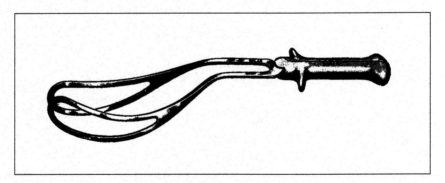

FIG. 1–3. Hawks-Dennen forceps with perineal curve for axis traction.

DeWees Forceps

The general configuration of the DeWees instrument is of a spread shank Simpson type. It has a French lock with a wing nut screw device to tighten the blades on the fetal skull. The traction bar is dropped by an extension attached to one handle so that axis traction is automatic (Figure 1–4).

Other similar examples of a Simpson-type instrument with attachments for axis traction that may be available are the Lobstein-Tarnier and the Good forceps. In addition to being cumbersome, these instruments were all designed for difficult, higher-level forceps procedures that should probably be avoided.

Mann Forceps

The instrument developed by J. Mann in 1956 (not his earlier instrument) employs rigid blades and parallel shanks. The blades

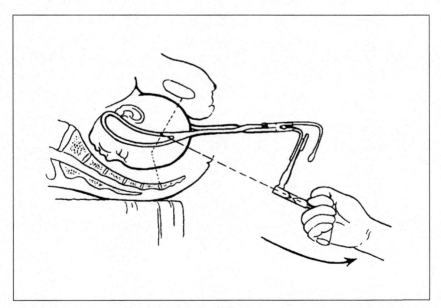

FIG. 1–4. Instrumental axis traction with DeWees forceps.

are connected with a wedge-shaped sliding lock that permits the blades to slide to different depths into the pelvis to adjust for asynclitism. The instrument is claimed to automatically adjust itself as the asynclitism disappears during rotation. Simultaneously, the shanks remain parallel while adjusting to heads of different sizes by locking at varying distances from each other. A bar attaches to the lock, serving as a handle for rotation and axis traction. The relatively straight pelvic curve permits application in any position of the occiput while minimizing compression. Rotation and traction may be accomplished without reapplication of the instrument.

Miseo Forceps

Representing another attempt to develop the universal obstetric forceps is the instrument reported by A. Miseo in 1956. This employs adjacent shanks to which the blades articulate at a split universal joint. The anterior blade is also hinged to allow application similar to that of the anterior blade of the Barton forceps. The hinge position and pressure to grasp the head can be adjusted with a turn knob in the handle. The ball-and-socket universal joint can be rotated in any plane or direction in the socket formed by the union of the proximal shanks. The joint can be locked and made rigid at any appropriate time. The thin blades are moderately fenestrated, and the pelvic curve has been eliminated from them.

The forceps can be applied in any position of the occiput, and application in the transverse is aided by the hinged anterior blade. Compression is minimized. After rotation and during descent, the universal joint can be unlocked to permit the head to follow the path of least resistance while axis traction is applied. No reapplication should be necessary.

Laufe Forceps

The new obstetric forceps described by L. Laufe in 1956 ingeniously incorporates features of the Kielland (see Chapter 5, "Special Instruments") and the Barton forceps, incorporating the advantages of both in a single instrument. Superficially, the Laufe forceps are similar to the Kielland instrument in length, handles, and sliding lock. The blade is longer and wider but symmetrical, lacking the Kielland's slight reverse curve in the shanks. The shank on the handle without the lock is hinged behind the blade, allowing an application similar to that of the anterior blade of the Barton forceps. After application, the hinge can be locked at the shank, thus providing a rigid instrument.

Divergent Forceps

An unusual instrument is the divergent outlet forceps as introduced by L. Laufe in 1968. The shanks are of the Elliot type, and the blades have a Luikart type of indented fenestration (see Chapter 2, "Classical Instruments"). There is a perineal curve without a pronounced pelvic curve. The blades are joined by a pivot lock at the end of the shanks. There are no handles; instead, finger grips for traction are located on the same side of the lock as its respective blade. Because no crossed first-class lever exists, compression of the fetal head by force transmitted from handle compression is not possible. Traction on the finger grips applies negative (divergent) force on the skull due to the physics of this arrangement. This somewhat reduces compression of the head.

Other instruments, such as the Leff forceps and the Shute forceps, of ingenious, inventive, and thoughtful design, have appeared. Perhaps undeservedly, they have not attracted wide acceptance and distribution.

CHAPTER 2

Forceps Classification According to Station of Head in Pelvis

*S*ince early in the 20th century, forceps categorization has been difficult, confused, and controversial. This has been due in part to problems with nomenclature and uncertainty in the application of terminology. The adjectives *floating, unengaged, high, mid, low–mid-, low, outlet, elective,* and *prophylactic* all have been used to describe types of forceps deliveries. Each could have meant different things to different operators, although some terms were almost synonymous.

Definitions

The American College of Obstetricians and Gynecologists (ACOG) issued its classification of outlet forceps, midforceps, and high forceps in 1988 and again in 2000. The ACOG defines *station* according to the level of the leading bony point of the fetal head in centimeters at or below the level of the maternal ischial spines (0–5 cm) (see box).

The ACOG definition is essentially a four-level classification that covers only those categories for which there can be a valid or, as with midforceps, a potential use in modern obstetrics. It is obvious that, when the leading bony point is at the inlet, a higher category than midforceps is inferred, although it is not an acceptable procedure. Criteria for types of forceps deliveries are shown in the box.

Definitions of Forceps Deliveries

1. **Station:** The relationship of the estimated distance, in centimeters, between the leading bony portion of the fetal head and the level of the maternal ischial spines. In classifying midforceps procedures, the level of engagement of the fetal head must be stated as precisely as possible. Engagement of the vertex occurs when the biparietal diameter has passed through the pelvic inlet and is clinically diagnosed when the level of the leading bony portion of the fetal head is at or below the level of the maternal ischial spines (0–5 cm).

2. **Outlet forceps:** The application of forceps when a) the scalp is visible at the introitus without separating the labia, b) the fetal skull has reached the pelvic floor, c) the sagittal suture is in the anteroposterior diameter or in the right or left occiput anterior or posterior position, and d) the fetal head is at or on the perineum. According to this definition, rotation cannot exceed 45 degrees. There is no difference in perinatal outcome when deliveries involving the use of outlet forceps are compared with similar spontaneous deliveries, and there are no data to support the concept that rotating the head on the pelvic floor 45 degrees or less increases morbidity. Forceps delivery under these conditions may be desirable to shorten the second stage of labor.

3. **Low forceps:** The application of forceps when the leading point of the fetal skull is at station +2 cm or more and not on the pelvic floor. Low forceps have two subdivisions: a) rotation 45 degrees or less (eg, left or right occiput anterior to occiput anterior, left or right occiput posterior to occiput posterior), and b) rotation more than 45 degrees.

4. **Midforceps:** The application of forceps when the fetal head is engaged but the leading point of the skull is above station +2 cm. Under very unusual circumstances, such as the sudden onset of severe fetal or maternal compromise, application of forceps above station +2 cm may be attempted while simultaneously initiating preparations for a cesarean delivery in the event the forceps maneuver is unsuccessful. Under no circumstances, however, should forceps be applied to an unengaged presenting part or when the cervix is not completely dilated.

Criteria for Types of Forceps Deliveries

Outlet forceps

1. Scalp is visible at the introitus without separating labia.
2. Fetal skull has reached pelvic floor.
3. Sagittal suture is in anteroposterior diameter or right or left occiput anterior or posterior position.
4. Fetal head is at or on perineum.
5. Rotation does not exceed 45 degrees.

Low forceps

Leading point of fetal skull is at station ≥+2 cm and not on the pelvic floor.

Rotation is 45 degrees or less (left or right occiput anterior to occiput anterior, or left or right occiput posterior to occiput posterior).

Rotation is greater than 45 degrees.

Midforceps

Station is above +2 cm but head is engaged.

High forceps

Not included in classification.

American College of Obstetricians and Gynecologists. Operative vaginal delivery. ACOG Practice Bulletin 17. Washington, DC: ACOG, 2000.

Another way of viewing the pelvis is to divide it into four planes (Figure 2–1) as follows: The plane of the inlet is bounded by the sacral promontory and the upper, inner border of the symphysis. The plane of greatest pelvic dimension extends between the middle of the inner border of the symphysis and the junction of the fused second and third sacral vertebrae, having crossed the obturator foramen. The plane of least pelvic dimension is bounded anteroposteriorly by the lower, inner border of the symphysis and the sacrococcygeal joint and laterally by the ischial spines. The plane of the outlet, quadrilateral in shape, is bounded by the sacrococcygeal joint posteriorly, the ischial tuberosities laterally, and the inferior border of the symphysis anteriorly.

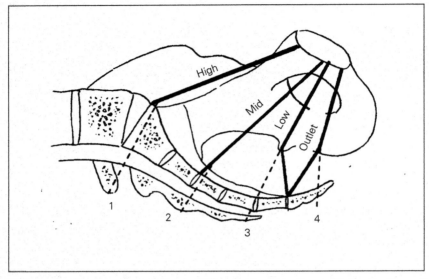

FIG. 2–1. The four major planes of the pelvis are 1) plane of inlet, 2) plane of greatest dimensions, 3) plane of least pelvic dimensions, and 4) plane of outlet.

A larger infant obviously has a longer distance to travel between the leading bony point and the biparietal diameter than does the smaller head of an infant weighing a kilogram less. There is also a greater tendency for molding to occur with a larger head. Because extreme molding lengthens the long axis of the head, the biparietal diameter is at a correspondingly greater distance from the leading point (Figure 2–2). The estimation of this distance is of the greatest importance because the biparietal diameter is the widest diameter of the fetal head that must pass through the maternal pelvis, and its level designates the true station of the head. With marked molding, in cases with the leading point on the perineum, the biparietal diameter may be at or above the ischial spines. What is often thought to be an easy outlet forceps delivery is later proved to be a difficult delivery of a head at low station or even midstation. Faulty attitudes, such as various degrees of extension of the head, including the extremes of brow and face presentation, and the abnormal attitude of asynclitism, influence the level of the biparietal diameter with relation to the leading point.

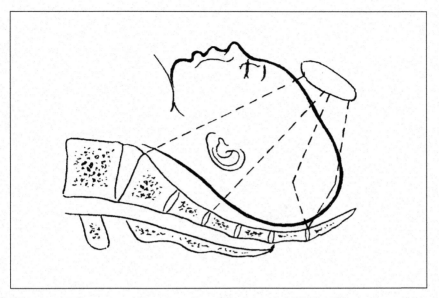

FIG. 2–2. Extreme molding in mid-occiput posterior presentation.

In extensions of the head, the biparietal diameter is farther from the leading point than in normal occipital presentations (Figure 2–3). The greater the extension, the more the variation. In asynclitism, either the anterior or the posterior parietal bone is presenting (Figure 2–4). Therefore, one extremity of the biparietal diameter is considerably lower than the other. The actual station of the head depends on the level of the "pivot point," which is the midpoint of the biparietal diameter. The location of this point must be judged by the degree of asynclitism and the level of the leading point. The more asynclitic the head, the more one is apt to consider the head at a lower level than is the case.

Clinically, this is more frequent in anterior asynclitism with the anterior parietal bone well under the symphysis and the hollow of the sacrum being empty. The degree of asynclitism can best be determined by the shape and location of the sagittal suture. The greater the asynclitism, the more the shape of the sagittal suture changes from a straight line toward the shape of the letter "U." With the anterior parietal bone presenting, the "U" is upright. In a poste-

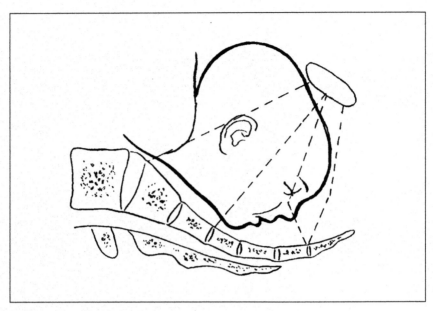

FIG. 2–3. High posterior chin.

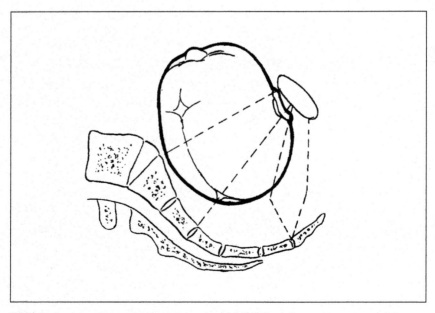

FIG. 2–4. Anterior parietal presentation, high left occiput transverse position.

rior parietal bone presentation, or posterior asynclitism, the "U" is inverted.

Deformities of the pelvis may predispose to and accentuate molding, extensions, and asynclitism. These deformities may involve any of the major planes of the pelvis and consequently affect the accuracy of the diagnosis of station.

Molding at the inlet is common in small gynecoid and android pelves, especially with posterior positions of the occiput. Asynclitism and extensions, even to the degree of face presentation, are frequently found in platypelloid pelves. With the head arrested at this level, the common mistake is to consider the head engaged when, in reality, the biparietal diameter is above the inlet.

Deformities of the plane of greatest pelvic dimensions, or the midplane, are accompanied by factors similar to those of the inlet and affect molding, extensions, and asynclitism. A transverse contraction in the anthropoid and android types frequently leads to a posterior position with more than average molding. A contracted anteroposterior diameter due to a straight sacrum or a forward-jutting sacral vertebra leads to extension and asynclitism. Hence, most of these cases should be classed as high forceps instead of midforceps because the biparietal diameter is usually at the inlet. This knowledge should influence the operator to avoid the dangerous higher-station procedures.

The greatest percentage of dystocias occur in the plane of least pelvic dimensions, which is the plane of the ischial spines. The android pelvis presents the most difficulty at this level. Here the molding is accentuated and may be so extreme that the leading point touches the perineum when the biparietal diameter is still above the ischial spines. The common error in diagnosis in such cases is to label the operation low forceps rather than midforceps.

Deformity of the plane of the outlet, particularly with a funnel pelvis, predisposes to posterior positions and excessive molding. Here again, if the diagnosis of station is made by the leading bony point alone, the delivery will be classed lower than the actual classification.

Because it may be difficult to determine the exact level of the biparietal diameter, it is important that the phrase *at the spines* is correctly understood. When a leading bony point is at the spines, it has reached a plane that includes the ischial spines laterally and the sacrococcygeal junction posteriorly. In such a situation, the hollow of the sacrum is nearly filled by the head. A common error is, upon feeling the fetal head in the anterior part of the pelvis, to consider the vertex at the spines without investigating further to determine whether the hollow of the sacrum is empty. The difference may be between a head that is in midpelvis and one that is high or unengaged. On occasion, with complicated cases, an erect lateral X-ray study can be a valuable diagnostic tool. The exact level of the biparietal diameter can be determined, and it may show a previously unrecognized deformity of the sacrum to be the cause of dystocia.

In the average case, it can be assumed that the biparietal diameter is located at a certain level, depending on the level of the leading bony point, as has been indicated. In cases with extreme molding or abnormal attitudes, and in deformed pelves predisposing to those conditions, the biparietal diameter automatically should be placed at least at the next higher plane.

Visual evidence of the fetal scalp at the perineum does not necessarily mean an easy outlet forceps delivery. Without a systematized classification, there is a great void between the outlet forceps, in which the head is visible, and the midforceps, which may be anything from the easiest procedure to a complicated delivery of a head at the inlet. This is one reason why the true midforceps operation has fallen into discredit.

Many studies have been published concerning the results of operative vaginal deliveries. The terms *outlet* and *low* have been used interchangeably in many instances. Despite the problems of nomenclature, operator bias, varying skill levels, differing indications, presence of monitoring, length of follow-up, and so forth, some general agreement has been reached. Early investigators considered the outlet, or low forceps, procedure to be preferable to spontaneous delivery. The National Institute of Neurological Disorders and Stroke's Collaborative Perinatal Project tended to agree with the earlier studies. This large-cohort, prospective, controlled study measured many parameters, with a 4-year follow-up. Later studies agree with the safety of the low (or outlet) forceps procedure. Several, in fact, again suggest results superior to those of spontaneous delivery.

The case for midforceps is more confusing. Data from the Collaborative Perinatal Project have been interpreted to support the opposing view of forceps protagonists and antagonists. Friedman and associates analyzed the data and showed small but statistically significant adverse long-term effects after midforceps delivery compared with spontaneous or low forceps delivery. Unfortunately, the risk factors (anesthesia, dystocia, distress) prompting the operative intervention were not documented, nor were midforceps results compared with those of cesarean delivery. In this study and others, it is unreasonable to compare the results of indicated midforceps delivery to those of spontaneous delivery. Generally, the only possible alternative is cesarean delivery.

Prerequisites for Forceps Deliveries

The indications for obstetric forceps may be either maternal or fetal. Maternal indications include maternal exhaustion, failure of labor to progress, or bleeding. In cardiac or pulmonary disease, a shortened second stage of labor may be indicated. Similarly, a history of spontaneous pneumothorax, detached retina, and so forth, would contraindicate bearing down.

Fetal indications include signs of distress, malposition (including the aftercoming head), or low birth weight (but not including a very-low-birth-weight infant weighing less than 1,000 g). In the past, 2 hours of the second stage of labor was considered a fetal indication. It has been shown that, in monitored fetuses, prolonged labor is not specifically associated with fetal depression or morbidity. Thus, one can be more relaxed concerning arbitrary time limits in the second stage. Cases should be individualized and evaluated to determine causes of labor disorders.

Elective or prophylactic forceps delivery, as advocated by DeLee, is no longer considered to be an indication. The prerequisites for a forceps delivery are of vital importance and should be emphasized.

They are as follows:

- The head must be engaged.
- The cervix must be fully dilated and retracted.
- The exact position of the head should be determined.
- The type of pelvis should be known.
- Appropriate anesthesia should be in effect.
- Adequate facilities and supportive elements should be available.
- The operator should have knowledge of the instruments, their use, and the complications that can arise.

Engagement

An unengaged head is considered to be a contraindication for a forceps delivery in all cases. The risk to both mother and fetus makes it unwarranted to attempt such a procedure.

Engagement is determined by the passage of the biparietal diameter through the plane of the inlet. Generally, it is accomplished when the leading bony point of the skull has reached the ischial spines, although extensive molding can give a misleading diagnosis by the unwary. The station of the head is marked and recorded as plus or minus centimeters of deviation below or above the ischial spines on palpation of the leading bony point.

Cervix

The cervix must be fully dilated and retracted. Should a lip of unretracted cervix be caught between the toe of the instrument and the fetal head, marked obstruction to rotation or descent of the head will be encountered. In addition, the risk of cervical laceration is great. There is no place in modern obstetrics for manual dilation of the cervix with the head under instrumental traction or for cervical incisions.

Position

The position of the head must be correctly diagnosed to achieve correct application and proper traction with the forceps. Most heads should be delivered in the occiput anterior (OA) position with an accurate application of the forceps. This reduces the effort necessary for delivery and lessens the risk of injury. Heads not in the OA position are rotated to OA either manually or instrumentally. The risk of injury is increased when the position is misdiagnosed, followed by an incorrect application of the forceps and improper traction. Not infrequently, the diagnosis of position is difficult to make. Continued practice and constant alertness are important factors in maintaining a high percentage of correct diagnoses. This problem may be simplified if attention is directed to the sutures rather than to the size and shape of a fontanelle, which often may be distorted or obscured by molding or caput formation. Three sutures, the two lambdoidals joined by the sagittal, forming the shape of the letter "Y," indicate the posterior fontanelle. An inverted "Y" to the left indicates a left occiput posterior presentation, an oblique upright "Y" to the patient's right indicates a right occiput anterior presentation, and a horizontal "Y" to the patient's left indicates a left occiput transverse presentation (Figure 2–5). In case of doubt, the sagittal suture should be traced to its opposite end. Identification of the anterior fontanelle is more readily made because it is formed by the junction of four lines meeting in the form of a cross. These lines are the two halves of the coronal suture meeting the sagittal and the frontal sutures.

Occasionally, on tracing the sagittal suture throughout its length, it will be found to be curved like the letter "U," with its most dependent portion closer to the sacrum than to the symphysis and with each fontanelle in an anterior quadrant of the pelvis. This should be recognized as an anterior parietal presentation caused by anterior asynclitism (Figure 2–6). Thus, what was originally thought to be an anterior position of the head—because the posterior fontanelle was found in an anterior quadrant—now will be diagnosed as a transverse position, rather than a left occiput anterior presentation.

Less frequently, the opposite situation will be found. In posterior asynclitism (Figure 2–7), the posterior parietal bone presents with the inverted "U" of the sagittal suture closer to the symphysis than

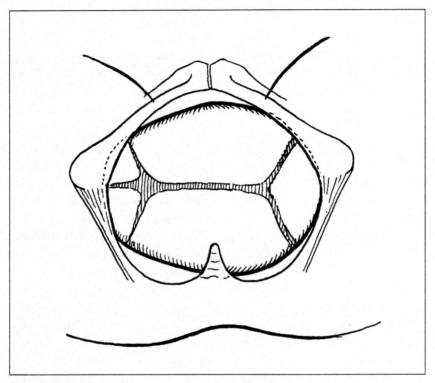

FIG. 2–5. Left occiput transverse presentation with normal synclitism.

to the sacrum and its extremities dipping into the posterior quadrants. This is likewise a transverse position and usually is found in a flat pelvis with an unengaged head.

If only one end of the sagittal suture can be felt and is thought to terminate in the posterior fontanelle, a check may be made. By sweeping the examining fingers over the supposed occipital bone from one side of the "Y" to the other (the presumed two halves of the lambdoidal suture), another suture line, which is a continuation of the sagittal suture, may be felt dividing the intervening space. If so, it makes a fourth line leading to the same point and is therefore the frontal suture leading into the anterior fontanelle. If doubt persists, the posterior ear may be palpated to establish the exact position

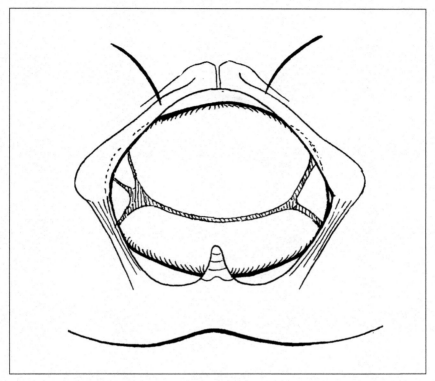

FIG. 2–6. Left occiput transverse presentation. The anterior parietal presentation is due to anterior asynclitism.

of the occiput. However, this procedure is reserved as a last resort because of the risk of displacement and backward rotation of the head. This risk is lessened if the operator has a small hand.

Although it has been said that a displaced head will come down again, unfortunately, this does not always occur, at least not in as favorable a position. Many of the technical difficulties of a forceps delivery may be avoided by not displacing the head. Occasionally, these difficulties are so great as to force the operator to abandon further attempts at forceps delivery in favor of some other procedure originally considered not indicated or more hazardous.

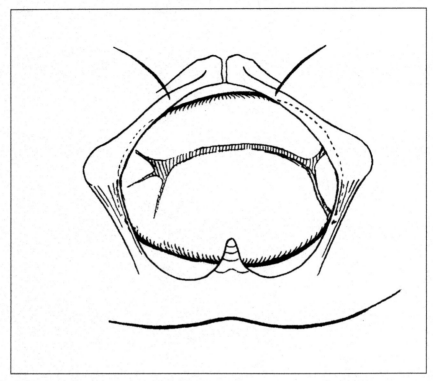

FIG. 2–7. Left occiput transverse presentation. The posterior parietal presentation is due to posterior asynclitism.

Pelvic Evaluation

The importance of the clinical evaluation of the pelvis for adequacy in the fetopelvic relationship should not be underestimated. Routine antepartum and intrapartum pelvic evaluation is advised but becomes particularly necessary with the development of an arrest pattern. An obstetrician with a reasonable concept of pelvic architecture has a prognostic advantage in anticipating and avoiding certain pitfalls in practice. Pelvic contractures are associated with abnormalities of dilatation and descent, fetal malposition, dystocia, and, obviously, operative obstetrics. Cephalopelvic disproportion, a contraindication to forceps procedures, must be ruled out. The indications for forceps procedures change depending on pelvic type and relative disproportion.

Although antepartum clinical estimation of fetal weight is a notoriously inaccurate art, it gains importance when pelvic evaluation indicates a potential inadequacy. Ultrasound evaluation of fetal size can aid in predicting a problem between a specific fetus and the pelvis that it must traverse.

The use of radiographic pelvimetry has greatly decreased over recent years. Although this is due in part to concern over the effects of radiation, there is also some lack of significance of the information gained with vertex presentations. The clinician can easily evaluate the outlet and midpelvis for configuration and obstetric import. The inlet and upper straits of the pelvis are naturally better evaluated with radiographic techniques, but frequently this is not necessary. Nonengagement of the biparietal diameter removes the inlet as a significant factor, in that a contraindication to operative vaginal delivery would exist.

Simple illustrations of the significance of the pelvis are numerous. A posttrauma, fixed, anteriorly angled coccyx may require fracture to remove obstruction to descent of the head. A history of childhood bony injury or back deformity can result in asymmetrical pelvic development and unusual diameters. Shortened anteroposterior diameters are associated with a higher incidence of shoulder dystocia, particularly with a prolonged second stage of labor and midpelvic delivery. These and other examples demonstrate that pelvic evaluation is important in obstetric management.

Anesthesia

Appropriate anesthesia is indicated for any forceps procedure, particularly when it is more than an outlet classification. Although reports have been published praising the safety and cost-effectiveness of a local anesthetic in the perineal body, this is felt to be far less than adequate for other than emergency situations. Minimum anesthesia is a good pudendal block. Many experienced operators find this procedure difficult and often inadequate. More preferable would be a conduction anesthesia, such as low spinal or epidural. Under certain circumstances, a brief general anesthesia or even nitrous oxide analgesia may be effectively employed.

The association between regional anesthesia and the need for forceps delivery is well documented. Prolonged labor and a significant increase in malpositions have been reported. Anesthesia expertise, particularly the use of segmental blocking epidural techniques, appears to obviate the problem.

Facilities

Adequate facilities and support personnel must be present. Although the simplest forceps operations may be undertaken in a birthing-room environment, the optimum conditions of a delivery room are usually advisable. In addition to the requirements as stated in ACOG's *Guidelines for Perinatal Care*, the operator should have at least level I ultrasound scanning available. In current obstetric practice, the use of postpartum cord pH determination, particularly in other than routine forceps procedures, is advisable. This, of course, is in addition to careful antepartum fetal and maternal monitoring.

In a situation in which a forceps procedure (or cesarean delivery) is indicated for fetal status, the presence of a person skilled in newborn resuscitation and treatment is mandatory. The skill and acumen of the obstetrician can be negated by inadequate care of a previously depressed infant.

Instruments

A knowledge of the types of instruments and their advantages, disadvantages, technique, and potential complications is necessary for proper choice and use of obstetric forceps. The instruments may generally be divided into two types: classical and special. Classical types comprise instruments that follow a style of construction and use that has been accepted as standard for years. Special types comprise more recently developed instruments that differ markedly from classical instruments in their principles of construction and technique of use. Some instruments have special advantages under certain conditions, whereas others are definitely contraindicated. Some fit the shape of molded heads; others, round heads. With some, a more accurate application can be obtained with less manipulation. Others give a better line of traction.

The classical instrument consists of two blades, each of which is connected to a handle by a shank. The blade may be fenestrated, solid, or solid with an indented fenestration. It is connected to the shank at an angle that corresponds to the curve of the pelvis. In addition to the pelvic curve, the blade has a lateral curve, known as the *cephalic curve*, corresponding to the side of the fetal head. The tip of the blade is the *toe*, and the portion of the blade that is attached to the shank at the posterior lip of the fenestration is the *heel*. At or near the junction of the handle and the shank is the *lock*. Originally, forceps had no locks, but as the modern instrument passed through its various stages of development there appeared fixed locks, semifixed locks, set screw locks, and crossbar locks. Almost all of the commonly available classical instruments in the United States employ the English lock. With this type of lock, each blade contains a slot into which the shank of the opposite blade fits. In the French lock, one blade contains a pin that fits in a notch on the opposite blade.

Classical Instruments

The type of classical instrument is determined mainly by its shank. There are two types of the classical instrument.

Elliot Type

The Elliot-type forceps (Figure 2–8) have overlapping shanks that impart a short, rounder cephalic curve to the blades. Due to the overlapping shanks, the blades must curve widely in order to attain a distance between them necessary to accommodate a fetal head with a biparietal diameter of about 9.5 cm. This bulging at the heels results in a rounder cephalic curve, making the Elliot-type forceps the instrument of choice for application to round, unmolded heads. The Elliot and the Tucker-McLane, and its modification by Luikart, are examples of the Elliot type of classical forceps.

Simpson Type

The Simpson-type forceps (see Figure 2–8) have parallel, separated shanks that result in a long, tapering cephalic curve. This type of cephalic curve makes the blade fit better on a longer, molded head.

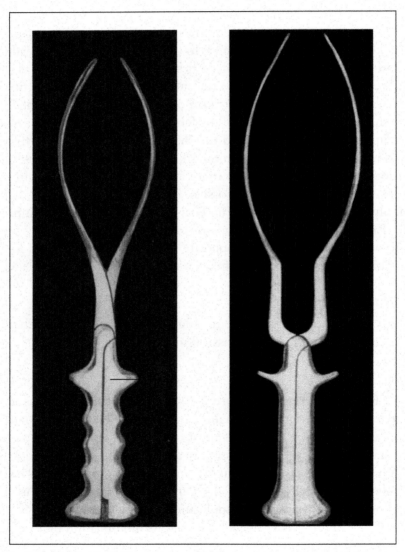

FIG. 2–8. Elliot (left) and DeLee-Simpson (right) forceps.

The Simpson, DeLee, Irving, and Hawks-Dennen forceps are examples of the Simpson type.

Special Instruments

Special forceps types include a number of instruments that employ different mechanical concepts. They are designed to have certain advantages in various clinical situations. The best known of these are the Kielland and the Piper forceps.

Complications

The complications associated with forceps use can be maternal and fetal. Maternal problems involve mainly trauma to soft tissue, including uterine, cervical, and vaginal lacerations; hematomas; bladder or urethral injuries; and episiotomy extensions. All of these complications have been reported with spontaneous delivery. Their frequency is greater with operative delivery, and their severity tends to vary inversely with the skill and judgment of the operator.

Related fetal injuries include transient facial forceps marks, bruising, lacerations, cephalohematomas, and facial nerve injuries. Less commonly, skull fracture and intracranial hemorrhage, potentially with falx or tentorial laceration, are reported. Again, these injuries have been seen with spontaneous delivery, though with a lower incidence, thus placing the onus on the operator. The more major problems generally indicate an injudicious use of the instrument.

CHAPTER 3

Technique

C orrect application of the forceps before traction is applied
is mandatory. All applications must be cephalic, that is, in
relation to the fetal head rather than to the maternal
pelvis. The so called "pelvic application" has no place in
modern obstetrics.

In a true cephalic application, the blades fit the head as evenly as
possible. Thus, the place of application of the blade and the shape of
the head must be considered. The blades should lie evenly against
the side of the head, reaching to and beyond the malar eminences,
symmetrically covering the space between the orbits and the ears
(Figures 3–1 and 3–2). There should be no extra pressure at any one
point. A correct application prevents injury to the head because the
blades fit the head accurately and pressure is evenly distributed. The
pressure is applied to the least vulnerable areas and is transmitted
symmetrically to the normally symmetrical intracranial structures.
Disruption of the falx cerebri or tentorium with intracranial hemorrhage is a risk when force is transmitted to an asymmetrical application, such as a brow-mastoid application.

Correct application allows the operator to know the exact attitude
of the head. Knowing the direction of the long axis of the head
should ensure descent in the proper attitude of flexion, minimizing the force necessary and decreasing trauma to maternal or fetal
structures.

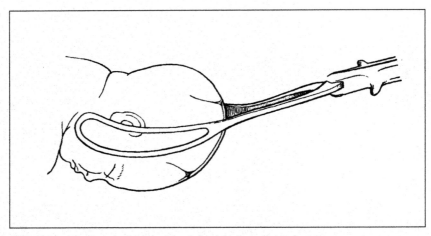

FIG. 3–1. True cephalic (biparietal, bimalar) application.

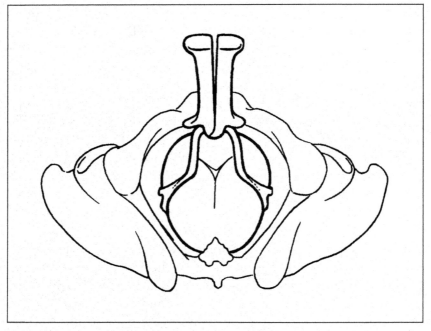

FIG. 3–2. Correct application according to the three checks (described under "Application in Left Occiput Anterior Presentation").

Technique of Application

The patient should be in the lithotomy position with appropriate preparation and draping. As previously noted, with rare exception, adequate anesthesia should be in effect. The bladder should not be distended.

A vaginal examination is performed, and if membranes are intact, they are ruptured. Station, position, and attitude of the fetal head are determined. During the examination, station should be maintained if possible because the higher the head the more complicated the operation.

The blades are identified by holding them locked with the pelvic curve up, directed toward the patient in the position in which they will be when applied to the sides of the head (Figure 3–3). The left hand of the operator grasps the handle of the left blade, and the right hand grasps the handle of the right blade.

There are four cardinal points to remember when the occiput is in the anterior position. The left blade, held in the left hand, is inserted into the left side of the pelvis in front of the left ear of the fetus. The cardinal points shift to the right when dealing with the right blade. It is also important to remember that in all left-sided positions of the occiput, the left ear is posterior; in right-sided positions, the right ear is posterior. In posterior positions, the posterior ear is on the opposite side of the pelvis from that of the corresponding anterior position; that is, in a left occiput posterior position, the left, or posterior, ear is on the right side.

With the sagittal suture in the anterior–posterior diameter, the left blade is applied first. This facilitates locking of the handles after application of the right blade, because the lock is usually on the left. With the sagittal suture in an oblique diameter of the pelvis, the posterior blade (the left blade for left occiput anterior [LOA] presentation and the right blade for right occiput anterior [ROA] presentation) is applied first. By using the posterior blade technique, a splint is provided for the head, which tends to keep it in its anterior position and prevents its backward rotation to the transverse, or even the posterior, position during the application of the anterior blade. This

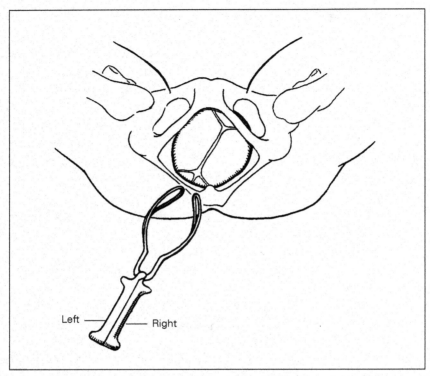

FIG. 3–3. Orientation for left occiput anterior presentation.

advantage far outweighs the slight disadvantage of the necessity of crossing the handles to accomplish locking the forceps in the ROA position.

Application in Left Occiput Anterior Presentation

In an LOA presentation, the left ear is posterior; therefore, the posterior blade is the left blade, the handle of which fits the operator's left hand. The posterior blade is introduced into the left side of the pelvis, in front of the left ear.

Temporarily, after discarding the right blade, the operator stands with his or her back toward the patient's right knee, holding the handle of the blade in his or her left hand by the precision grip. The blade's pelvic curve is directed downward and its cephalic curve is directed inward toward the vulva, as the plane of the shank is kept perpendicular to the floor. Maintenance of this position directs the blade properly on its intended course along the curved plane of the head and the left posterior side of the pelvis to its intended place in front of the left ear. Using any other position of the blade starts it moving in the wrong direction. The middle and index fingers of the operator's right hand are then inserted into the vagina opposite the posterior, or left, parietal bone to guide the toe of the blade along the side of the head. The right thumb is placed against the heel of the blade as the cephalic curve of the blade is laid against the curve of the skull. The force necessary to carry the blade into the vagina to its proper place is applied mainly with the thumb rather than the left hand at the handle. The left hand merely guides the handle downward over an arc, first outward toward the right thigh, then inward toward the midline, as the blade enters the vagina (Figure 3–4). Force applied at the handle may be uncontrolled and unconsciously increased if resistance is met, thereby causing damage. The force exerted by the thumb at the heel is limited, and because it is applied directly on the blade, it is less likely to deflect the blade from its proper course.

Once the blade has been applied, if the pressure of the pelvis is not sufficient to hold it in place, an assistant holds it exactly as placed. In an LOA presentation, the plane of the handle should be parallel to the left oblique diameter of the pelvis, at right angles to the sagittal suture, or approximately coinciding with a line connecting the numerals 10 and 4 on the dial of an imaginary clock.

A mistake often made by beginners is to change the handle so that it is parallel to the floor. This is an incorrect application unless the head has also rotated to the occiput anterior (OA) position, with the sagittal suture perpendicular to the horizontal and coinciding with a line connecting 12 and 6 on the dial of a clock.

In applying the second, or anterior, blade, the four cardinal points shift from left to right, and the operator changes position so that his or her back is now toward the patient's left knee. The right blade,

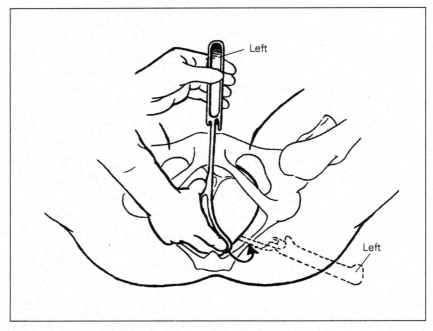

FIG. 3–4. Introduction of left (posterior) blade in left occiput anterior presentation.

held in the right hand, is applied similarly, except that the toe is inserted anteriorly on the right side at a higher level so that it is adjacent to the anterior frontal bone. If the right blade is inserted posteriorly, as the left blade was, it must be guided around the brow to the anterior, or right, ear by the operator's middle and index fingers, which have replaced the thumb at the heel of the blade. As this is done, the fenestration may catch on a corner of the brow, causing the head to rotate back to a left occiput transverse position. Thus, the good application of the first blade is lost. The result is often the undesirable brow-mastoid application. The arc described by the handle of the right blade is longer in its downward component to carry the toe into the anterior quadrant over the right malar eminence.

When the right blade is in place, the handles are locked (Figure 3–5). The left blade is not moved; because it was applied first, it is more apt to be in the correct position, and the right blade is adjusted

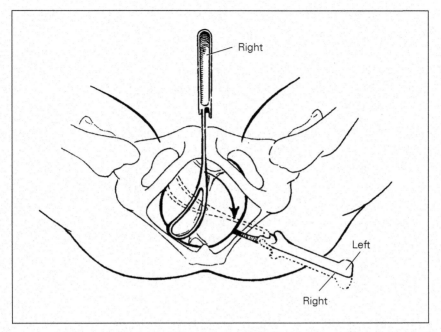

FIG. 3–5. Introduction of right (anterior) blade and locking of handles in left occiput anterior presentation.

to fit it. If the handles do not lock easily or if they diverge widely when locked, the application is incorrect. Usually, this is due to incomplete rotation of the anterior blade beyond the brow on the cheek and a short application. This is overcome by lowering the handle after unlocking it and elevating the blade by exerting upward pressure on the heel of the right blade with the middle and index fingers of the left hand. This carries it farther up into the pelvis and around to the side of the head. If this maneuver is not successful, the forceps should be removed. The position of the head should be carefully checked, and if it is found to be the same, the application is repeated.

After the handles are locked satisfactorily, the application is checked. This is done in three ways (see Figure 3–2):

1. The *posterior fontanelle* should be located midway between the sides of the blades and one finger's breadth above the plane of the shanks.

2. The *sagittal suture* should be perpendicular to the plane of the shanks throughout its length.
3. The *fenestrations* of the blades should barely be felt, if at all. It should be possible to insert no more than the tip of a finger between them and the head. The amount of fenestration felt on each side should be equal.

Unless these conditions are fulfilled, the application is not a true cephalic or biparietal bimalar application, and readjustment of the blades is therefore necessary. This may be done without removing them. Readjustment is more easily accomplished after the head is rotated counterclockwise with the forceps, without traction, until the sagittal suture is in the OA position. Attempts at readjustment before rotation of the occiput to the anterior position often result in upward displacement of the head, backward rotation to left occiput transverse position, and no improvement in the application (Figure 3–6).

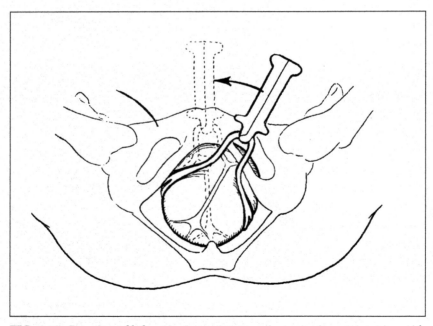

FIG. 3–6. Rotation of left occiput anterior to occiput anterior presentation with Simpson-type forceps preliminary to traction.

If the posterior fontanelle is more than one finger's breadth above the plane of the shanks (first check of application), correction is very easily made. The handles are unlocked, elevated one at a time to the required level, and then relocked. If traction is applied without this correction, the result is the same as traction on a deflexed head. The pivot point of the head is above the center of the blades. Traction causes further extension of the head. This requires more force, with the accompanying risk of injury.

If the posterior fontanelle is less than a finger's breadth above, or even below, the plane of the shanks, the pivot point of the head is below the center of the blades. The application is in the overflexed attitude, and the toes of the blades are too far forward on the cheeks. Traction causes further flexion of the head. Correction is made by unlocking the handles and depressing or sinking the handles against the perineum one at a time until the shanks are at the desired level below the posterior fontanelle.

When the sagittal suture runs obliquely to the plane of the shanks (second check of application), it signifies a brow-mastoid application. Many of the milder degrees of this type of application are not recognized unless the examining finger is passed along the entire length of the sagittal suture to determine its ultimate direction.

Correction is made by unlocking the handles and adjusting one blade at a time, usually the posterior one first, without removing them. The handle is moved slightly away from the midline to move the toe of the blade away from the head. Pressure is then exerted on the heel of the blade as pressure is applied in the opposite direction on the handle in order to shift the blade until the plane of the shank is perpendicular to the sagittal suture. The other blade is then adjusted in the same manner, but in the opposite direction, until its shank is also perpendicular to the sagittal suture. The handles are then relocked and the position checked. Occasionally, the entire maneuver may have to be repeated if the result is not at first satisfactory.

If more than one-half inch of fenestration is felt below the head (third check of application), it signifies a short application. The toe of the blade is not anchored well beyond the malar eminence. This may cause the forceps to slip during traction. If the operator is not prepared, the blades may come entirely off the head, causing deep lacerations. In the correction, the unlocked blades are carried, one at a time, farther up into the pelvis until the fenestration cannot be felt below the head. The handles are then depressed and locked. After a final check of the application and anterior rotation, the next step is traction.

Application in Right Occiput Anterior Presentation

The technique of forceps application in ROA presentation is similar to that in LOA, except that the order of application of the blades is reversed. In the ROA position, the posterior blade is the right blade and is applied first. It is held in the right hand and inserted posteriorly into the right side of the pelvis in front of the right ear (Figure 3–7). The left blade, held in the left hand, is then applied anteriorly

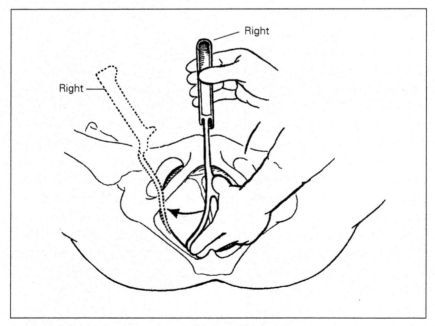

FIG. 3–7. Introduction of right (posterior) blade in right occiput anterior presentation.

to the left side of the pelvis in front of the left ear (Figure 3–8). Because the standard lock is on the shank of the left blade, it will be necessary to separate the handles and cross the upper, or left, handle under that of the lower, or right, handle in order to lock them (Figure 3–9). After clockwise rotation to the OA position (Figure 3–10), checking the application, and making the necessary readjustments, traction is begun.

Traction

The ultimate and dominant function of the obstetric forceps is traction in order to accomplish descent of the head in the birth canal. The only other primary function that is now considered is rotation in order to bring the head to the most favorable position for descent. In the past, forceps were used under certain circumstances as levers

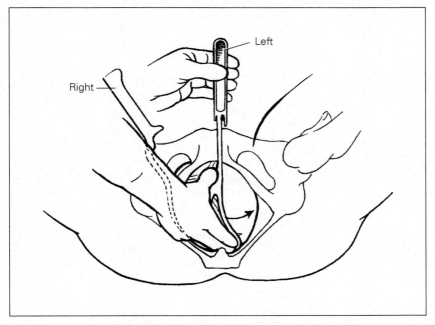

FIG. 3–8. Introduction of left (anterior) blade in right occiput anterior presentation.

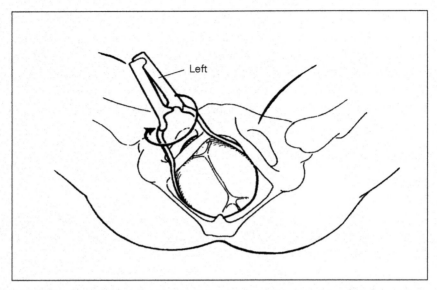

FIG. 3–9. Crossing handles (left under right) for locking in right occiput anteri-or presentation.

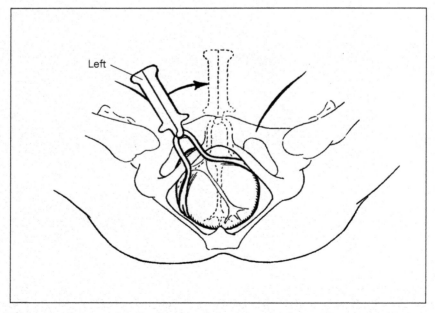

FIG. 3–10. Rotation of right occiput anterior to occiput anterior presentation with Simpson-type forceps preliminary to traction.

to wedge the head into and through the pelvis. Because maternal structures served as the fulcrum, serious injury to mother and fetus was common. When destructive operations were performed, forceps were used as compressors, even perforators.

Compression is an effect rather than a function of forceps, and great pains must be taken to minimize it. As DeLee eloquently stated: "The accoucheur should always remember, when working with forceps, that he or she has a child's brain in the grasp of a powerful vise, and that only the greatest care and gentleness will save its wonderfully delicate structure from injury."

The student of forceps technique is impressed by compressive force when he or she places his or her fist between the toes of the instrument and squeezes the handles with the opposite hand. This often pictured (and used) technique employs the principles of a first-class lever and applies compressive force to the skull. When force is applied at the finger guards, much closer to the fulcrum at the adjacent lock, very little compressive force is applied between the toes and the cephalic curve.

Strain gauge measurements of tractive and compressive forces to the skull during forceps deliveries have been performed. The maximum compressive force is less than 5 pounds (2.25 kg) when traction is applied at the finger guards. This is considerably less than that surmised by earlier authors. Compression is not directly proportional to tractive force and shows little change after application. Compression helps to maintain position of the instrument on the head during traction with all instruments and is supplied by maternal structures, namely, the pelvic walls and intervening soft tissues.

In the case of any position other than OA, rotation of the head to the OA position is usually necessary before traction is applied. Depending on the pelvic configuration and capacity, rotation usually is easily performed with the biparietal diameter close to the plane of greatest pelvic dimensions. It can, of course, frequently be performed at a lower level.

If one thinks in the analogous terms of an egg in a tube, rotation is most readily accomplished with the long axis of the egg aligned with the long axis of the tube. An off-center rotation results in friction and resistance. Similarly, the fetal head must rotate along its long axis, roughly perpendicular to the suboccipital–bregmatic plane.

When the forceps are correctly applied, a line connecting the toes of the instrument should meet the line representing the long axis of the head. Any rotation of the instrument should be performed with the toes describing an arc that is as small as possible, thus maintaining the long axis of the head in the same direction. Ideally, of course, that direction is perpendicular to the plane of the pelvis at the level of the biparietal diameter. Here the operator must think first in terms of the toes of the instrument and their movement. Secondarily, he or she must consider the effective widest transverse diameter of the head that must be moved—the biparietal diameter and its assumed level in the pelvis.

A most important consideration related to rotation of the head is the fact that classical forceps lose their pelvic curvature as they turn away from the anterior position. With a 90-degree rotation from OA to occiput transverse, the pelvic curve becomes a lateral curve and the instrument no longer can correct for the direction of the birth canal. Consequently, the level of the handles must be lowered relative to the horizontal in an amount that increases with the degree of rotation away from OA. Failure in this respect is reflected in difficulty with the procedure and will leave the telltale sign of increased marking of the anterior cheek of the infant.

Traction is divided into two elements, both of which must be considered: direction and amount. Traction should always be applied in the axis of the pelvis. A picture of the pelvic curve as a stovepipe with an elbow at its lower end should be kept in mind when applying traction. Force is applied in a plane perpendicular to the plane of the pelvis at which the head is stationed. Because the widest point of the head—the biparietal diameter—is being moved, it is the station of that point that must be considered. The higher the head, the lower from the horizontal is the line of traction. As the head descends, the line of traction moves forward in a curved line following the curve of the sacrum and then upward through the outlet. The pelvic curve of the classical instrument directs the handles in a plane obliquely anterior to the plane of the pelvis at which the head is stationed. Therefore, traction in the direction of the handles results in force being wasted against the symphysis and the possibility of accompanying injury and little or no advancement of the head (Figure 3–11).

To apply force in the plane of least resistance, that is, the axis of the pelvis, the axis traction principle must be employed. This may be accomplished manually. One hand grasps the shanks and the other hand grasps the handles at the finger guards. Force is exerted in two directions: downward with the hand on the shanks and outward with the hand on the handles. If the operator is standing, a downward push with the palm of the hand on the shanks results in the Pajot maneuver. For those who prefer the seated position, the fingers of the hand on the shanks pull vertically downward in the Saxtorph maneuver (Figure 3–12). The resultant force, or vector, is in a direc-

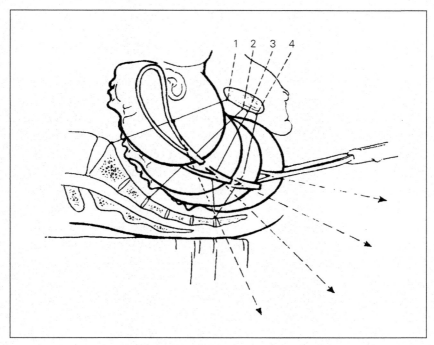

FIG. 3–11. Line of axis traction (perpendicular to the plane of the pelvis at which the head is stationed) at different planes of the pelvis: 1) high, 2) mid, 3) low, and 4) outlet.

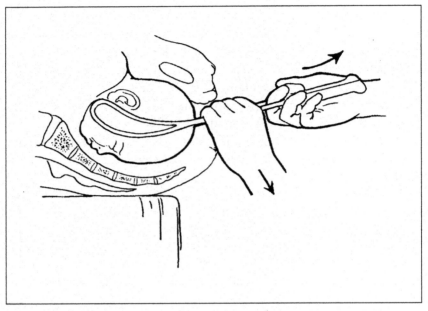

FIG. 3–12. Manual method of axis traction—the Pajot-Saxtorph maneuver.

tion determined by the relative strengths of the outward and downward forces. This method is followed by various degrees of success depending on the skill of the operator and the station of the head. The higher the head, the more difficult it is to achieve axis traction by the manual method. Axis traction is best obtained with some form of axis traction attachment, permitting traction to be applied in a lower plane that approaches that of the pelvic axis (Figure 3–13).

The amount of tractive force should be the least possible to accomplish the necessary descent. It is important for the operator to remember that the procedure is not a contest of strength. Rather, it requires thought, skill, and finesse in following the planes of least resistance.

Studies have shown that the maximum pull along the proper axis should never exceed 45 pounds (20.25 kg) in a primipara and 30 pounds (13.5 kg) in a multipara. Most deliveries are accomplished with less force. Judging this amount of pull becomes relatively easy if one experiments with a traction-measuring instrument or even

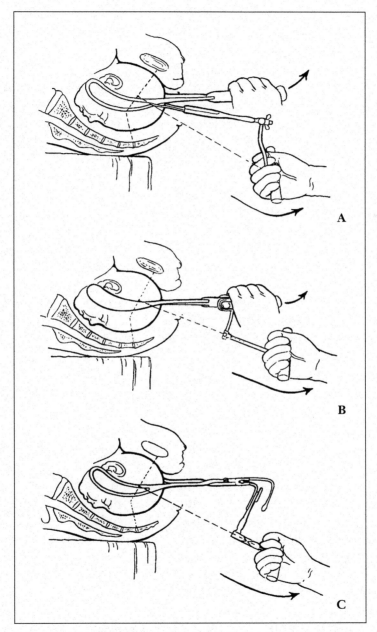

FIG. 3–13. Instrumental axis traction: **A.** Irving, **B.** Tucker-McLane, solid blades with Bill handle, and **C.** DeWees.

orthopedic weights in a bag hung over a pulley. An experienced operator working with a mannequin can supply appropriate counter-traction to the efforts of the student.

As with the vectored traction direction, the amount of vectored force is difficult to deduce from muscle strength applied outward and downward on the instrument. This is the reason for the often-advised use of an instrumental axis traction in other than the simplest cases. Although an axis traction forceps such as the DeWees may be used, the simpler use of the Bill axis traction handle on the finger guards can suffice. Similarly, special instruments with reverse or mechanically variable pelvic curve may be employed. In these instances, the vectored force becomes automatic for direction and amount when pull is applied to the handle. Another important consideration is that less total muscle power is required and the operator can appear more relaxed to nonmedical observers in the delivery suite.

Traction may be applied from either the sitting or the standing position according to the operator's preference. Some prefer the seated position because of greater ease in gaining axis traction. The seat should be directly in front of the patient. It may be adjustable, but it must be stable. If standing, the operator adjusts position so that the dominant hand can be used for traction. Posture should be erect and the feet in a "fighter's stance" to maintain balance in case of sudden advancement or slippage of the forceps. For control, the arms should never be extended. Rather, the elbows should be close to the sides so that the operator uses shoulder and arm muscles instead of leaning backward using back and leg muscles. If the instrument has no axis traction attachment, the handles rest in the upturned palm of the dominant hand. The shanks separate the middle and index fingers that grasp the finger guards in the Elliot type of forceps. If a Simpson type is used, the middle finger occupies the space between the shanks and the adjacent fingers grasp the finger guards. Compression of the fetal head from squeezing of the handles is thus avoided.

The nondominant hand grasps the shanks close to the vulva from below, if sitting, or from above, if standing. This hand becomes the fulcrum hand for the Saxtorph or Pajot maneuver, exerting downward pressure.

The traction hand applies traction outward in the direction of the handles, and the fulcrum hand pulls or pushes directly toward the floor. The result of these two forces tends toward axis traction. As the head distends the perineum and the occiput passes under the symphysis, the direction of the pull changes to follow a curved plane forward and upward. This change in direction is carried out gradually and only during traction, following the plane of least resistance. Observation of the relationship between the upper edge of the blade and the scalp adjacent to it can help in determining the direction of pull. The head tends to keep its long axis close to the axis of the pelvis, held by pressure from the maternal structures. If the operator elevates the forceps too soon, the head cannot extend and the scalp appears to sink in relation to the upper edge of the blade. Conversely, late elevation of the instrument during traction results in the scalp rising as the head extends. The operator can then adjust the direction of pull accordingly.

Traction is made with a steady pull that is gradually increased in intensity, sustained for a definite interval, and then gradually relaxed. Under appropriate circumstances, and ideally, the timing should coincide with a uterine contraction and bearing down by the patient. The amount of force necessary for a gradual advance of the head and the number of tractions necessary for delivery vary with each patient. Careful monitoring of the fetal heart should be maintained during rest periods between contractions. Monitoring equipment may be quickly removed when delivery is imminent.

Under no circumstances is force greater than that delivered by the arms and shoulders to be used. Anecdotal stories of an operator bracing his feet on the table to increase traction are to be deplored.

Episiotomy may be performed before traction or when the perineum is being distended by the head. Late episiotomy has the advantages of having the rectum pushed posteriorly out of the field and of less bleeding due to compression of the vessels in the distended perineum. Early episiotomy results in the need for less traction force, thus avoiding early injury to soft parts in traction. The risk of a "buttonhole" rectal injury from episiotomy scissors can be prevented by using two spread fingers to depress the anterior rectum away from the incision site. Episiotomy if performed, should be median except in rare circumstances, such as very unusual anatomy, previous fistula repair, or, possibly, Crohn's disease.

As the head is extended over the perineum, the forceps handles are elevated by the fulcrum hand, leaving the traction hand free to perform a Ritgen maneuver. To protect against sulcus lacerations, the handles should not be elevated higher than about 45 degrees above the horizontal. At this time, the operator's fingers, protected by a sterile towel, catch the chin through the perineum behind the anus, preventing the head from receding. The uncovered thumb of the same hand is placed directly against the occiput to prevent a precipitous advance of the head during the removal of the blades.

The blades are removed by a reversal of the motion used in applying them. The right blade is removed first. After the blades are unlocked, the handle of the right blade is carried over an arc toward the left groin and up to the symphysis. This is performed with the hand that is not occupied with the Ritgen maneuver. As the handle is elevated, it is rotated so that the blade emerges from the vagina across the occiput in a curved plane, with the cephalic curve of the blade following the curve of the head (Figure 3–14). The left blade is removed with the same hand in a similar manner, toward the right side.

If resistance is encountered in removing the right blade, the left may be removed first. If both blades tend to stick, traction is not made on the handle because of the risk of injury to both the mother and the fetus from forcible extraction. If necessary due to resistance, it is acceptable to deliver the head with one or both blades in situ. After removal of the forceps, the head is delivered by the modified Ritgen maneuver. Restitution is completed manually. The shoulders and body are delivered in the usual manner.

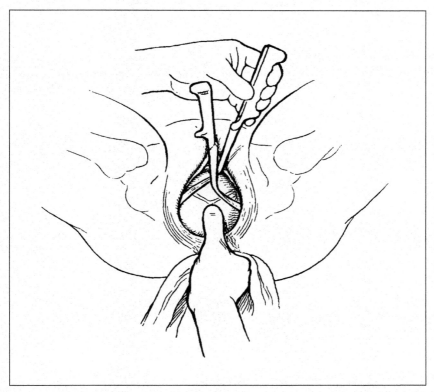

FIG. 3–14. Removal of forceps while head is controlled by the modified Ritgen maneuver.

CHAPTER 4

Other Positions

*I*n the left occiput transverse (LOT) position, it is often difficult to get a good application with the classical instrument. It is even more difficult in the right occiput transverse (ROT) position, because the handles must be crossed to lock them and an accurate application may be lost by this maneuver. An alternative preferred by many obstetricians is the use of a special instrument such as the Kielland forceps. Before applying the blades, the operator may choose to rotate the head digitally or manually to the anterior position.

Digital and Manual Rotation

Left Occiput Transverse Presentation

Digital rotation, which is occasionally successful, can make the more complicated manual rotation maneuver unnecessary. Digital rotation may be used with or without anesthesia to supplement any rotational tendency evoked by the patient's bearing-down efforts. In digital rotation, the tips of the index and middle fingers of the right hand are placed in the anterior segment of the lambdoidal suture near the posterior fontanelle. The elevated edge of the anterior parietal bone offers resistance to the fingertips so that when a lifting motion is carried out, the occiput may be turned in a counterclockwise direction to the left occiput anterior (LOA) or even the occiput anterior (OA) position. The thumb may also be used with gentle downward

53

pressure more anteriorly on the parietal bone to aid this rotation. Counterpressure with the fundal hand tends to fix the head in the new position. If delivery is appropriate at this time, the two rotating fingers are slipped behind the posterior parietal bone to prevent backward rotation and act as a guide for the introduction of the left (posterior) blade.

If digital rotation is unsuccessful, the manual maneuver is used. The hand used in the rotation depends on the position of the head. In left-sided positions, rotation is accomplished with the right hand, because that is the hand used later to guide the introduction of the posterior, or left, blade. The four fingers of the right hand are introduced into the vagina behind the posterior parietal bone, with the palm up and the thumb over the anterior parietal bone. The head is grasped with the tips of the fingers and thumb. If the entire hand is introduced into the vagina, the head may be displaced or even disengaged. This should be avoided because the higher the head, the harder and more dangerous will be the operation. The head is flexed and rotated in a counterclockwise direction to the anterior position, or at least to the OA position (Figure 4–1). Simultaneously, the left hand is placed on the abdomen and pulls the back of the child toward the midline. When this has been accomplished, pressure is placed on the fundus to fix the head in the new position. To prevent the head from rotating back to its original position, only the thumb of the right hand is removed from the vagina, leaving the four fingers in place to splint the head and guide the introduction of the left blade in the usual manner (Figures 4–2 and 4–3).

After the left blade has been applied, an assistant holds the handle firmly, exerting a slight amount of force in the direction of the patient's left leg. This presses the toe of the blade against the fetus's left cheek and keeps the head in the anterior position. The right blade is introduced in the usual manner. This blade must be introduced high above the posterior frontal eminence to avoid this obstruction. The handle is moved toward the patient's left thigh to shift the toe slightly away from the obstructing anterior frontal eminence. The blade is then lifted with the middle and index fingers of the operator's left hand, which have replaced the thumb at the heel,

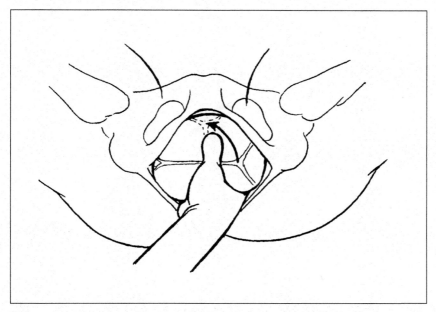

FIG. 4–1. Manual rotation from left occiput transverse to left occiput anterior presentation.

in order to bring it over the anterior parietal bone. If the fenestration catches on the frontal eminence, the head will rotate back to the LOT position and the result may be a brow-mastoid application. After the shanks are locked, the application is checked. If the head is in the LOA position, rotation to the anteroposterior (OA) diameter is completed and the necessary readjustments are made before traction is begun. If the application is unsatisfactory after two attempts at readjustment, both blades are removed, the position is checked, and the procedure is repeated.

Left Occiput Transverse Presentation

In ROT presentation, the left hand is the rotating and splinting hand. After rotation, the right, or posterior, blade is held in the right hand and inserted into the right side of the pelvis over the right ear. The left, or anterior, blade is held in the left hand and introduced high on the left side of the pelvis opposite the left ear in a similar

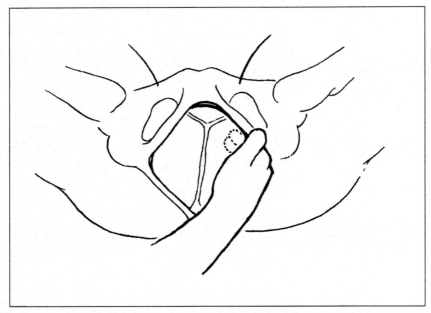

FIG. 4–2. Left occiput anterior presentation after manual rotation from left occiput transverse presentation. The fingers of the operator's right hand are in place, preventing backward rotation of the head. The operator's thumb is removed in preparation for the introduction of the posterior (left) blade.

manner as was the anterior blade in the LOT position. The handles must be crossed in order to lock them, because the lock is on the left shank. The head, if in the right occiput anterior position, is rotated without traction to the anterior–posterior diameter, the application is checked, the necessary readjustments are made, and traction and delivery are carried out in the usual manner.

In general, the station of the head indicates whether to attempt the digital or the manual maneuver. When the head is close to the plane of the outlet, the digital maneuver is chosen because there is insufficient room for the manual maneuver without displacement of the head. When the head is at a slightly higher station, the digital maneuver is less likely to be successful and there is room to try the manual maneuver without the necessity of the initial displacement of the head.

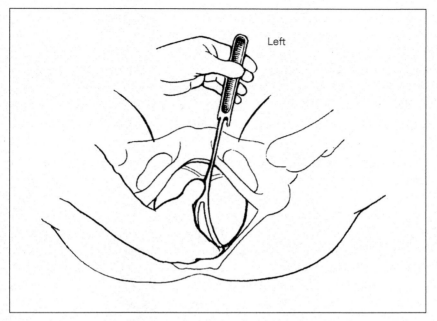

FIG. 4–3. Insertion of left blade (Simpson type) in application to left occiput anterior presentation after manual rotation from left occiput transverse presentation.

Instrumental Rotation

Left Occiput Transverse Presentation

An accurate application of forceps to the head in the transverse position is more difficult to accomplish than in the oblique position because the anterior blade has to be carried, or "wandered," over a longer arc around the face to the anterior ear directly under the symphysis. In doing this, the operator may meet more points of obstruction. When a proper application is accomplished, the plane of the shanks is directed toward the side on which the occiput lies, obliquely away from the midline of the long axis of the patient at an angle of about 50 degrees. The amount of deviation depends on the degree of the pelvic curve of the forceps and the position of the fetal head. The plane of the shanks deviates from the horizontal plane depending on the level of the biparietal diameter, because the instrumental pelvic curve is lost in a transverse application.

The wandering maneuver of applying the anterior blade to the transverse head is more easily accomplished with the Elliot type of forceps. Its rounder cephalic curve tends to offer less resistance than the Simpson as it is passed under the symphysis. The overlapping shanks also offer less resistance to rotation than the spread shanks of the Simpson-type instrument.

The left blade is introduced first, directly posteriorly instead of to the left side of the patient. Therefore, the approach differs from that of the anterior position, in that the plane of the shank is not perpendicular to the horizontal but runs obliquely to it in order to allow for the pelvic curve of the blade. The toe of the blade is directly posterior and the blade parallels the plane of the sacrum, the shank following obliquely to the plane of the sacrum. The blade hugs the head to avoid obstruction. As the blade enters the vagina, the handle is lowered until it reaches a point just below the horizontal, following the plane of least resistance. The fenestration should be only barely felt below the head. The angle made by the handle with the horizontal depends on the station of the head. "The higher the head, the lower the handle" (Figure 4–4).

The right blade is held in the right hand and introduced into the right side of the pelvis, high up under the ramus, because the brow is more anterior than in LOA presentation owing to the transverse position (Figure 4–5). The handle is then made to descend over an arc close to the left thigh as upward pressure is applied with the middle finger of the left hand to the heel of the blade (Figure 4–6). This maneuver throws the toe of the blade away from the anterior frontal eminence, wandering it around the head into place just in front of the anterior ear. As the handle of the wandering (right) blade approaches the handle of the posterior (left) blade, it will be found to be in a lower plane. In order to lock them, it will be necessary to elevate the handle of the right blade, causing it to slide farther up into the pelvis behind the symphysis until the handles meet. When locked, the handles lie in a plane obliquely to the left of the midline of the patient. This is necessary in order to bring the

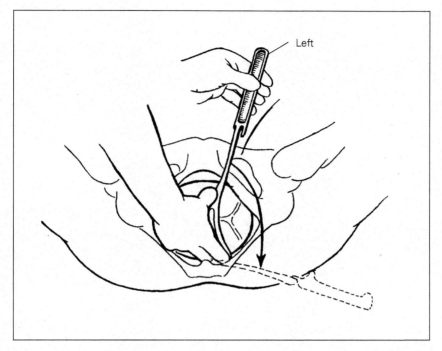

FIG. 4–4. Introduction of posterior (left) blade (Elliot type) for instrumental rotation of left occiput transverse to occiput anterior presentation.

plane of the shanks one finger's breadth medial to the posterior fontanelle.

In the instrumental rotation, the steps are as follows. To accomplish flexion, the handles are moved in an arc and then depressed. With slight compression on the handles to fix the blades on the head, the handles are moved toward the midline, far enough to correct the flexion attitude. The handles are then rotated upward in a wide, counterclockwise arc, consistent with the pelvic curve of the instrument (Figure 4–7). The object is to maintain a small arc with the toes of the blade, keeping the long axis of the head in the axis of the pelvis. As the 90-degree rotation is completed, the occiput comes to rest under the symphysis. The handles are depressed at completion to preserve or improve flexion, and the application is again checked. If necessary, the blades are readjusted before traction is

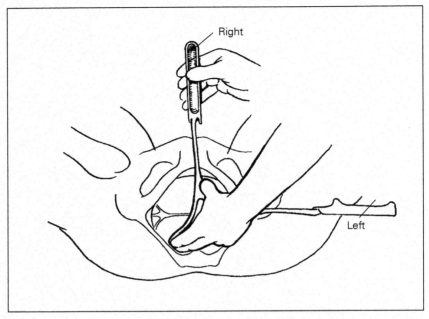

FIG. 4–5. Introduction of anterior (right) blade (Elliot type) for instrumental rotation of left occiput transverse to occiput anterior presentation.

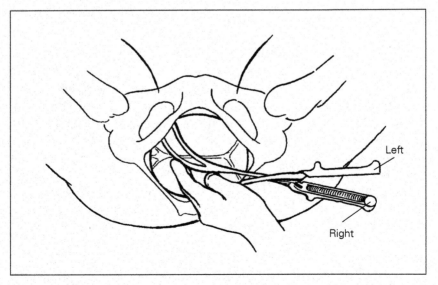

FIG. 4–6. "Wandering maneuver" of anterior (right) blade of Elliot-type forceps in application to left occiput transverse presentation.

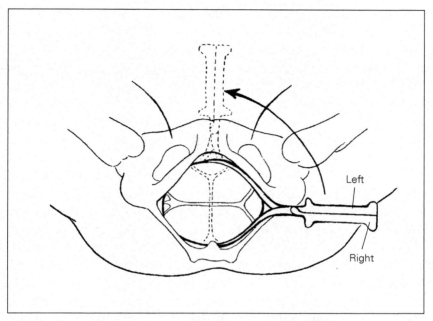

FIG. 4–7. Instrumental rotation of left occiput transverse to occiput anterior presentation.

applied in the axis of the pelvis. Traction is best performed with some form of axis traction instrument or attachment.

If the head will not rotate easily, it is probably because the handles are not being moved over a wide arc or because the head is extended. These situations may be corrected. The head may be arrested with a minor relative disproportion at the level of least pelvic dimension, that is, the ischial spines. In that instance, the head may require slight upward displacement so that rotation may be accomplished closer to the plane of greatest pelvic dimension.

If rotation remains difficult, the operator should reevaluate the pelvis, the fetal position, and the station. Repeated attempts at rotation are unwarranted and potentially dangerous.

Right Occiput Transverse Presentation

In ROT presentations, the right, or posterior, blade is introduced first. This is done by holding the right blade in the right hand and applying it directly posterior to the right ear. The force exerted to introduce the blade is made mainly by the thumb pressing against the heel. The handle descends toward the right thigh so that the shank will be one finger's breadth medial to the posterior fontanelle. This avoids an application in the extended attitude. The handle may be held in this position by an assistant while the left blade is introduced high on the left side and wandered anteriorly in the usual manner. In right-sided positions, the handles must be crossed in order to lock them. As this is done, the finger guard may interfere with the crossing, in which case one handle is pulled down while the other handle is pushed up, facilitating the crossing. A preliminary check of the application is made, and if it is found to be good, the head is flexed and rotated by carrying the handles clockwise over a wide arc to the anterior position. The application is then rechecked. Readjustments, which are frequently found to be necessary in this position, are made and extraction is completed in the usual manner. If the application is not satisfactory after attempts at readjustment, the blades are removed and, after the position is checked, they are reapplied.

Chapter 5

Special Instruments

Kielland Forceps

*I*n 1915, Christian Kielland of Norway presented his forceps to the obstetric world. Although originally intended for application to fetal heads in deep transverse arrest, the Kielland forceps is now used on heads in posterior presentations and, occasionally, in face and brow presentations. The instrument enjoys considerable popularity as a rotator in cases in which the occiput is not in one of the anterior quadrants of the pelvis. Some operators claim excellent results in elective low forceps use, and it has even been advocated as a substitute for Piper forceps to the aftercoming head.

In the past, the Kielland forceps was considered appropriate for heads arrested in the higher levels of the pelvis, although this was not its inventor's original intention. Currently, this type of higher-station forceps procedure is not generally considered justifiable in view of the reported increased incidence of poor fetal results. In addition, the incidence of failure with Kielland forceps is greater with higher stations of the head. Studies have indicated a greater neonatal morbidity and perinatal loss with Kielland rotation as compared with vaginal delivery. Vaginal delivery, however, is not an available alternative when operative delivery is indicated. When Kielland forceps results have been compared with those of cesarean delivery—a more relevant comparison—equal or superior results have been reported for the forceps operation. Moreover, results with Kielland forceps do not differ significantly from nonrotational forceps or manual rotation followed by forceps delivery. In the author's opinion, however, the Kielland procedure has a less traumatic "feel" and is preferable.*

Construction

The Kielland forceps has a slightly backward pelvic curve, giving the instrument a bayonet-like shape. It has overlapping shanks with an extra-long distance between the heels of the blades and the intersecting point of the shanks. The lock is a sliding one and is designed to correct for asynclitism. The inner surface of the blades is beveled to prevent injury to the fetal head. The knobs (or buttons) on each anterior surface of the finger guards are used to identify the anterior surface of the instrument and serve as a guide in the technique of application.

Advantages

The advantages of the Kielland forceps include the following aspects:

- A single accurate application without displacement of the head can be obtained by the inversion method because of the instrument's reverse pelvic curve.
- The sliding-lock principle permits adjustment of asynclitic heads and allows the handles to be locked at any level on the shank.
- A semi-axis traction pull is produced by the reverse pelvic curve.
- The beveled inner surface of the blades minimizes facial injury.
- The extra-long distance between the heels of the blades and the intersecting point of the shanks lengthens the posterior portion of the instrument's cephalic curve, accommodating heads of different shapes and sizes regardless of molding.
- The relatively straight design puts the shanks and handles close to the long axis of the fetal head, allowing the toes of the blades to describe a very small circle during rotation along the long axis.

---

*Outcomes associated with the use of Kielland forceps also are discussed in ACOG Practice Bulletin 17, "Operative Vaginal Delivery," June 2000.

Disadvantages

Disadvantages of the Kielland forceps have also been noted. In a flat pelvis with a high transverse arrest of a fetus in a posterior parietal presentation, the Kielland forceps are distinctly contraindicated. When applied to this position, the instrument provides no available pelvic curve or axis traction. The mechanism of a flat pelvis requires descent of the head in the transverse diameter. A straight or forward-jutting upper sacrum presents the same problem, regardless of the station of the head in transverse arrest. The head must be drawn well past the point of deformity, in the transverse position, before it can be rotated to the anterior position.

In a male-type pelvis with a funnel outlet and a low symphysis, the reverse pelvic curve of the Kielland forceps may cause injury to the posterior vaginal wall and perineum during extension. During the same maneuver, elevation of the handles may bring the portion of the forceps that connects the blades to the shanks in contact with the pubic rami, possibly resulting in a periostitis. These potential problems are of particular significance if the operator thinks in terms of a classical instrument, with its pronounced pelvic curve. Experimentation on a mannequin quickly demonstrates the location of the instrument's toes and shanks during extension. Some operators prefer to remove the Kielland forceps after rotation and some descent have been accomplished, substituting a suitable classical type of instrument with a good pelvic curve. They believe, probably without reason, that the Kielland forceps should be replaced with a better traction instrument for completion of the delivery.

Although the introduction of the Kielland forceps marked a great advance in obstetric surgery, it is not a panacea. It can be dangerous if not properly used, potentially resulting in perforation of the uterus, vesicovaginal fistula, perforation of the cul-de-sac, cervical and sulcus tears, and third- or fourth-degree laceration. All of these injuries can follow the use of any instrument, however, and some occur in spontaneous deliveries. The fault is not so much with the instrument as with the manner of its use.

Technique

The methods of application of Kielland forceps are listed here in the order of frequency of their indicated use:

1. Inversion is indicated for transverse and posterior presentations, except direct occiput posterior presentation, in most anthropoid and android pelves and in all gynecoid pelves. Contraindications are platypelloid pelvis, especially one with a posterior parietal presentation; straight or deformed sacrum that shortens the anterior–posterior diameter of the midpelvis; unavoidable resistance or obstruction to the use of this maneuver; a direct occiput posterior position; and a transverse position with an anterior parietal presentation well down in the pelvis.

2. Wandering is indicated for transverse positions when the inversion method meets resistance. Because the head usually is incompletely flexed, the anterior blade is wandered around the side of the face. Contraindications are the same as those for the inversion method.

   2A. Reverse wandering is used when the head is well flexed; the anterior blade is wandered around the side of the occiput, thereby avoiding resistance caused by the forehead.

3. Direct application is used for transverse positions in the outlet with an anterior parietal presentation. The anterior blade is inserted directly (not inverted) to the anterior cheek and ear, which often can be palpated behind the symphysis. The direct method is rarely used in anterior presentations because a classical type of forceps is preferable in those situations.

   3A. Upside-down direct application is used for direct occiput posterior presentations near the outlet. The blades are applied upside-down directly to the sides of the head. This method is used with caution on android and anthropoid pelves, some of which have insufficient room for anterior rotation of the occiput. Such cases may require delivery as an occiput posterior.

The standard method of application in most instances is the inversion method, which provides the main advantage of the Kielland forceps—namely, a single, accurate application without displacement. It can be accomplished without undue hazard because of the construction of the instrument.

The term *classical method*, instead of the more specific term *inversion method*, has crept into the literature and into case histories. This term is not favored because it has led to confusion, being misinterpreted as referring to the classical method used for applying a classical type of forceps. When referring to the Kielland forceps, it suggests the wandering method and not the standard procedure by inversion.

Left Occiput Transverse Presentation—Deep Transverse Arrest

Inverse ("Classical") Method of Application

Before the operative procedure is begun, the urinary bladder should be emptied. Performance of the procedure on other than a delivery table is not advised; birthing room facilities are generally inadequate. The patient must be positioned down toward the end of the table, buttocks slightly overhanging the edge. If not, difficulty may be encountered in application and rotation as the table edge prevents lowering of the handles perpendicular to the plane of the pelvis at the level of the biparietal diameter.

Because the Kielland is a special type of instrument, the technique used for classical instruments—applying the posterior blade first—is abandoned. Instead, the anterior blade is always applied first, preferably by Kielland's inversion method. In left-sided positions, the left ear is posterior and the right ear is anterior. This position requires the application of the right blade first. The blades are locked and held outside the pelvis, directed toward the patient in a position similar to that which they will assume when applied (Figure 5–1†). The knobs point in the direction of the occiput, toward the patient's left

† Figures 5–1 through 5–4 and Figures 5–12 through 5–17 depict application of the Kielland forceps with the biparietal diameter at the plane of the inlet. The transverse arrest as pictured would be a high forceps. The technique is no different at midforceps or low forceps levels.

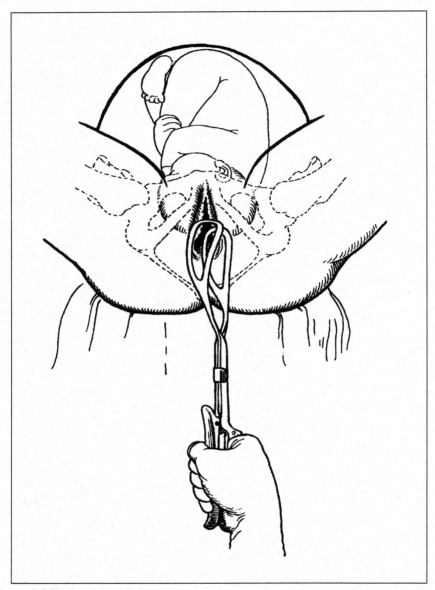

FIG. 5–1. Orientation. Position of Kielland forceps in left occiput transverse presentation.

leg, at 3 o'clock. The anterior blade is easily distinguished as the one on top and is found to be the right blade because there is no lock on its shank. This blade, after temporarily discarding the left blade, is held in an inverted position, with the inner surface of the cephalic curve facing upward and the shank 45 degrees above the horizontal.

The right blade, the handle of which is held in the right hand, rests in the palm of the left hand, the tips of the middle and index fingers of which are inserted under the symphysis, anterior to the head (Figure 5–2). The toe of the blade, guided by the operator's fingertips, is then passed directly under the symphysis. The cervix, when fully dilated and retracted, should not be palpable. If obstruction be met when the toe has passed the fingertips, gentle advancing pressure with a slight "pump handle" motion may be employed, feeling for the plane of least resistance. The object is to maintain the toe close to the head until the fenestration has disappeared from sight. Excessive force during this maneuver is ill advised.

By this time, the handle has been lowered in the midline to the level of the horizontal. When the heel of the blade has passed under

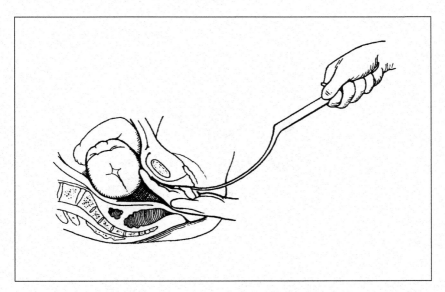

FIG. 5–2. Introduction of anterior (right) blade of Kielland forceps to anterior (right) ear in left occiput transverse presentation by the inversion method.

the symphysis, the handle has been further depressed to an angle of about 45 degrees below the horizontal, and the fenestration has reached its destination opposite the anterior cheek. The toe of the instrument may now be seen elevating the lower abdominal wall through the lower uterine segment. The elbow of the blade at the leading end of the shank should be close to the introitus, bringing a narrower diameter of the instrument between the head and the symphysis. The higher the head is in the pelvis, the lower the handle will be below the horizontal, and the further into the uterus the blade will have to be inserted (Figure 5–3).

Because the blade has been introduced in an inverted position, its cephalic curve is directed away from the head, toward the anterior wall of the uterus. The blade must now be rotated so that its cephalic curve will coincide with the curve of the head. The blade is rotated on its own axis *away* from the occiput, toward the midline and toward the knob. This maneuver is accomplished with the right hand grasping the handle and the thumb pressing against the side of

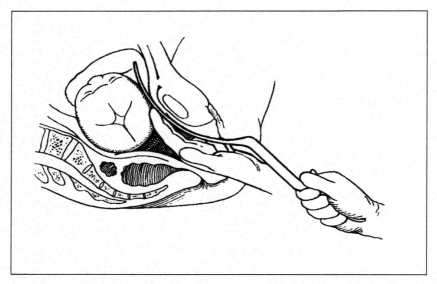

FIG. 5–3. Anterior (right) blade of Kielland forceps in place opposite the anterior (right) ear, with the forceps' cephalic curve directed away from the head, in left occiput transverse presentation.

the finger guard opposite the knob, turning it counterclockwise with a twist of the wrist over an arc of 180 degrees until the knob points toward 3 o'clock. As the rotation is being completed, the handle is depressed slightly in order to follow the plane of least resistance (Figure 5–4). If the blade is rotated in the wrong direction, that is, *toward* the occiput, the high point of the toe rubs against the anterior wall of the uterus and might cause damage.

Greater force is not used if resistance to rotation is encountered. In such instances, the blade may not be inside the cervix or, if it is inside the cervix, it may be either not far enough or too far inside the uterus. Resistance to both introduction and rotation of the blade may also be encountered in the presence of a low contraction ring. Introduction of the blade carries more risk than rotation because in rotation the beveled edge will not cut the uterus but will lift it away from the head. In contrast, during introduction, the toe could be forced through a thin lower uterine segment.

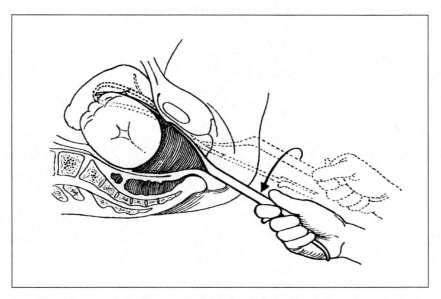

FIG. 5–4. Rotation of anterior (right) blade of Kielland forceps counterclockwise in left occiput transverse presentation so that the forceps cephalic curve will coincide with the curve of the head.

Wandering Method of Application

If it is not possible to rotate the anterior blade of the Kielland forceps after it is inside the uterus, the attempt to use the inversion method of application is abandoned. The operator then applies the anterior blade by the gliding, or wandering, maneuver, carrying it around the face to the anterior ear, as is done with the classical instrument (Figure 5–5). If the head is well flexed, interference often is encountered in wandering the blade around the side of the face. This may be avoided by reversing the maneuver and wandering the same blade, upside-down, around the side of the occiput (Figure 5–6). Some operators prefer to use the wandering method exclusively, in the belief that it is less hazardous than Kielland's inversion

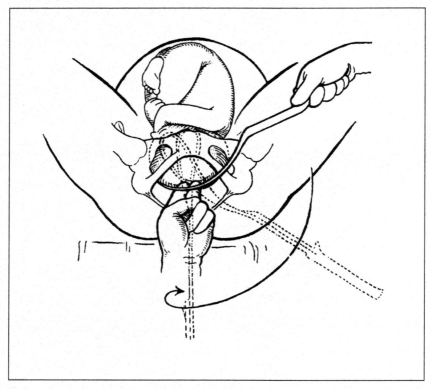

FIG. 5–5. "Wandering maneuver" for application of the anterior (right) blade of the Kielland forceps to the anterior (right) ear in left occiput transverse presentation.

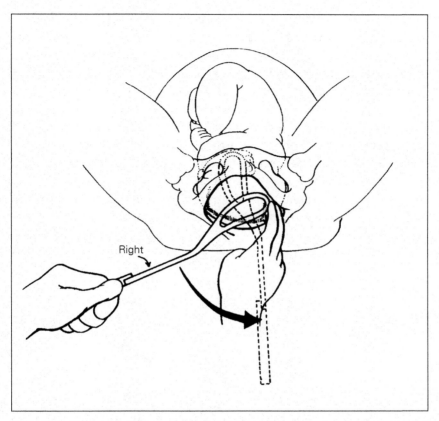

Right

FIG. 5–6. "Reverse wandering maneuver" for application of the anterior (right) blade of the Kielland forceps, held upside-down in the left hand, inserted to the left side of the pelvis, and wandered counterclockwise to the anterior (right) ear of fetus in left occiput transverse presentation with flexed head.

method. If the inversion method is not used, however, one encounters the same disadvantages accompanying the use of the wandering method with the classical instrument.

Direct Method of Application

Infrequently, the head is so low in the pelvis in the transverse position that it is difficult or even impossible to apply the anterior blade of the Kielland forceps by either the inversion or the wandering method. This situation is encountered when the head is near the outlet in the transverse position with an anterior parietal presentation. Because of the asynclitism and the depth of engagement, the anterior ear can be palpated vaginally just behind the symphysis. In such a scenario, a direct application is preferred.

In the direct application, the anterior blade—which is the right blade for a left occiput transverse (LOT) presentation and the left blade for a right occiput transverse (ROT) presentation—is applied directly under the symphysis to the anterior ear (Figure 5–7). The approach is made from below upward, the handle pointing toward the floor, below the edge of the table. The concave, beveled surface of the blade is in contact with the anterior parietal bone, and the toe is directed under the symphysis toward the anterior ear. With gen-

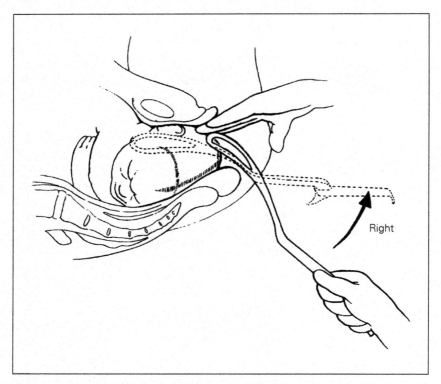

FIG. 5–7. Direct application of anterior (right) blade of Kielland forceps to anterior (right) ear of left occiput transverse presentation. The vertex is near the perineum, with marked anterior parietal presentation.

tle upward insertion, the blade slides up to the desired location on the anterior cheek.

Posterior Blade

After application of the anterior blade by the appropriate application technique, the posterior, or left, blade is introduced. The left blade is always introduced posteriorly between the shank of the anterior blade and the patient's right thigh, regardless of the method of application of the anterior blade. This technique obviates the necessity of crossing the handles in order to lock them. Guiding fingers, palm up, are introduced inside the vagina posterior to the head. The blade, with the cephalic curve up, is passed directly behind the head along the palmar surface of the guiding hand (Figure 5–8). Because of the obstruction that may be caused by the promontory, more difficulty may be encountered with the introduction of this blade than

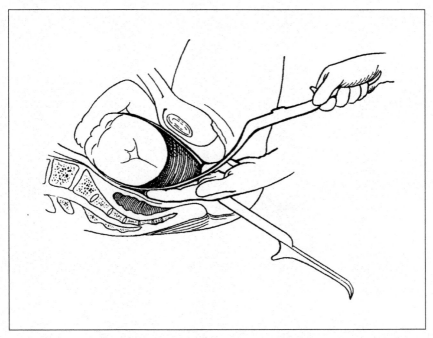

FIG. 5–8. Introduction of posterior (left) blade of Kielland forceps directly to the posterior (left) ear in left occiput transverse presentation.

with the anterior. If resistance is met, the handle of the posterior blade may be moved up and down, with a jiggling motion as it is inserted, in order to bring the toe inside the retracted cervix and keep it hugging the head. If resistance is met in the midline, the direction of the toe can be shifted slightly to either side of the midline to avoid an obstruction.

When the blade is opposite the posterior, or left, ear, the shanks are locked (Figure 5–9). The sliding lock permits this to be done at any level on the shank. One handle may be at a higher level than the other because an asynclitic application. Traction is made on the finger guard that is nearer the perineum. Simultaneously, pressure is applied in the opposite direction to the other finger guard until the handles are equalized, thus correcting the asynclitism. If the posterior blade cannot be inserted far enough to permit locking, the use of extra force should be avoided. Rather, downward traction on the handle of the anterior blade against the head should cause the latter to descend on the inclined plane of the cephalic curve of the posterior blade far enough to allow the handles to be locked. After a pre-

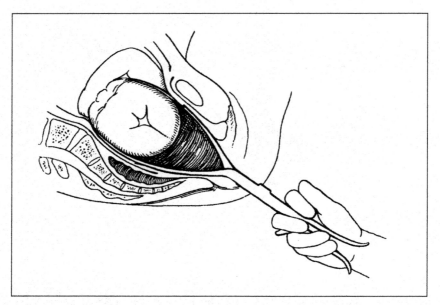

FIG. 5–9. Kielland forceps applied to left occiput transverse presentation.

liminary check of the application, the head is rotated counterclockwise 90 degrees to the occiput anterior position.

Rotation

Because of the reverse pelvic curve of the Kielland forceps, the instrument is rotated not over a wide arc but almost directly on the axis of the shanks, and the handles are depressed at the completion of the turn (Figure 5–10). The rotational force required should not be great. The novice is usually amazed that pressure from the thumb and index finger on the finger guards can easily accomplish most rotations. If visual control is not feasible during the procedure, the operator can use a finger resting on the scalp to check that the head is rotating with the forceps.

If resistance to rotation of the head is encountered in a normal pelvis, it is most commonly due to a failure to depress the handles to the proper level, that is, perpendicular to the plane of the pelvis at the level of the biparietal diameter. In this case, the operator should lower the handles for a higher biparietal diameter.

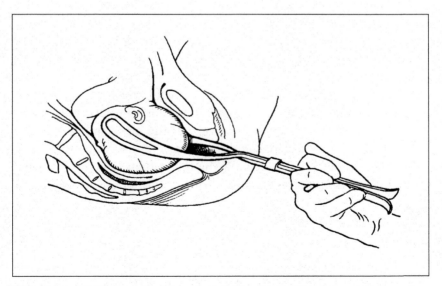

FIG. 5–10. Kielland application after counterclockwise rotation of left occiput transverse to occiput anterior presentation.

Extension of the head obstructs rotation along its long axis. Flexion is accomplished by readjustment of the forceps so that the plane of the shanks is within a finger's breadth anterior to the posterior fontanelle. The handles are then lightly compressed and carried to the midline and rotation can then be attempted.

On occasion, rotation at the level of application may be difficult. To bring the biparietal diameter to a different level in the pelvis, the operator should try downward traction for 1–2 cm rather than losing station. Should easy rotation be unsuccessful, the head should be displaced upward to a centimeter above its original station. This maneuver should bring the biparietal diameter well into the plane of greatest pelvic dimension, and rotation should proceed.[†]

If a situation is met in which rotation cannot be accomplished, the operator must eschew obstinacy and, particularly, the use of greater force. The forceps may be removed and the overall situation re-evaluated. Reapplication may then be tried.

Traction

After rotation has been completed, the application is rechecked, and if it is found to be correct, traction is begun. Traction, which is a backward pull in the direction of the handles, may be aided by the Saxtorph or Pajot maneuver. The finger guards are encircled by the middle and index fingers of the dominant hand, with the palm up (Figure 5–11).

Because the slight reverse pelvic curve of the Kielland forceps provides a semi-axis traction pull, the direction of traction is considerably lower than with classical forceps. If the biparietal diameter is in the plane of greatest pelvic dimension, the direction of traction should be about 45 degrees below the horizontal. Voluntary bearing down by the patient is always used to assist in traction, assuming this

---

[†]In earlier editions, the warning was given that "traction with the head in the transverse diameter of the inlet is contraindicated if the bulge of the anterior blade is above the symphysis, because it exerts force against the symphysis and the bladder." Because there is no present-day reason to use high forceps, this statement has become unnecessary. Similarly, displacement of the head to the inlet or higher, in order to accomplish rotation, is a dangerous procedure. Subsequent traction is on an unengaged head. The risk of such a procedure makes cesarean delivery the preferable route.

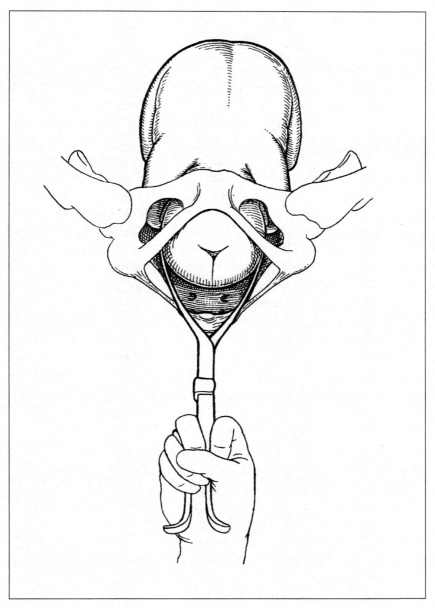

FIG. 5–11. Traction on occiput anterior presentation after anterior rotation with Kielland forceps.

is feasible. An episiotomy may be performed at an appropriate time. Lowering of the legs may give further relief of tension on the perineum.

As the posterior fontanelle is delivered, the forceps handles are gradually elevated to the horizontal during traction. The technique is similar to that use with classical instruments, except that it is important never to elevate the handles of the Kielland forceps above the horizontal. If this is done, the backward pelvic curve of the blade may cause a sulcus tear. To gain more extension, the operator may employ a special maneuver. Pressure is applied to the fundus by an assistant to keep the head from receding. The handles are unlocked and depressed, one at a time, toward the floor, so that the plane of the shanks is two or three fingers below the posterior fontanelle. The handles are then locked and elevated to the horizontal as slight traction is made. This maneuver causes extension of the head without digging the toes of the blades into the sulci. It may be repeated to gain the required extension for the performance of the Ritgen maneuver. The blades are then removed, taking the top, or right, blade off first, following the technique of the classical type of instrument. If difficulty is experienced in removing the blades, it is advisable, rather than using undue force, to deliver the head with one or both blades still in place.

Right Occiput Transverse Presentation

Because the left ear is anterior in an ROT position, the left blade, which is the anterior blade and has the lock on it, is applied first (Figure 5–12). The left blade is applied under the symphysis and into the uterus as already described (Figures 5–13 and 5–14). It is then rotated clockwise away from the occiput and toward the midline until the knob on the handle points toward the patient's right leg at 9 o'clock (Figure 5–15). The posterior blade is applied between the shank of the anterior blade and the right thigh, as is done in the LOT position (Figures 5–16 and 5–17). The head is rotated clockwise to the anterior position. The application is rechecked, and if it is found satisfactory, traction is applied and delivery is completed (Figure 5–18).

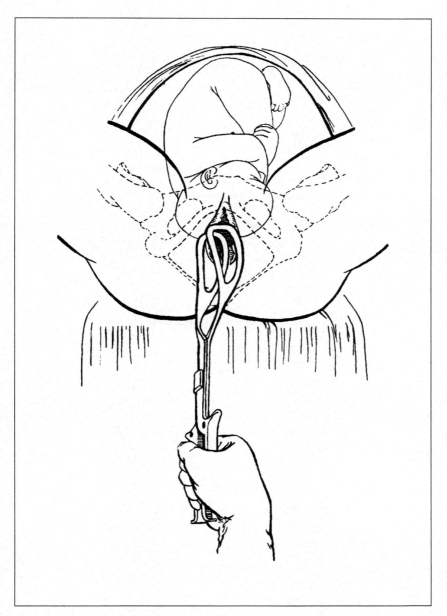

FIG. 5–12. Orientation for position of Kielland forceps in right occiput transverse presentation.

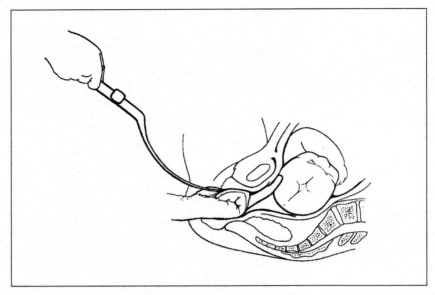

FIG. 5–13. Insertion of anterior (left) blade of Kielland forceps to anterior (left) ear of right occiput transverse presentation by the inversion method.

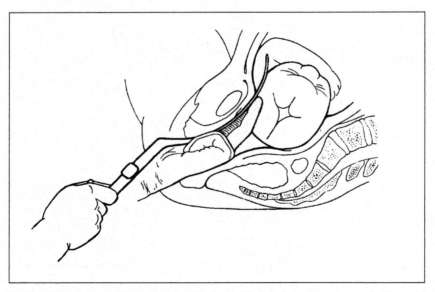

FIG. 5–14. Anterior (left) blade of Kielland forceps opposite anterior (left) ear of right occiput transverse presentation.

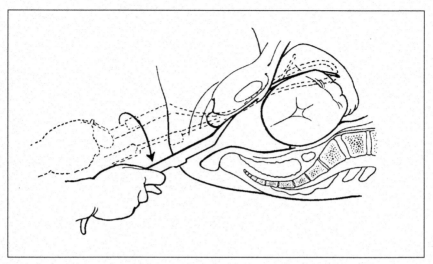

FIG. 5–15. Clockwise rotation in right occiput transverse presentation of anterior (left) blade of Kielland forceps so that its cephalic curve will coincide with the curve of the head.

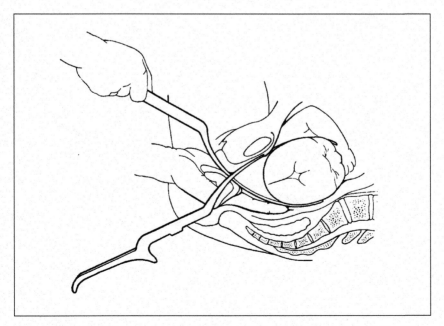

FIG. 5–16. Application of posterior (right) blade of Kielland forceps directly to posterior (right) ear in right occiput transverse presentation.

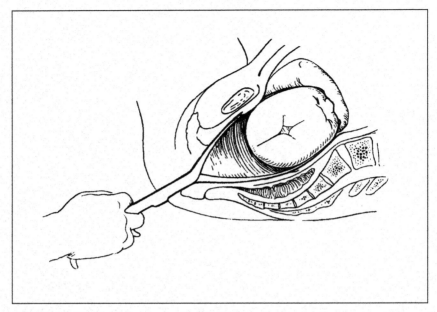

FIG. 5–17. Kielland forceps applied in right occiput transverse presentation.

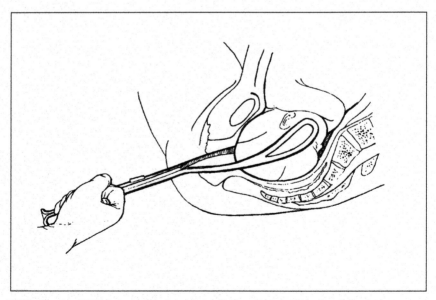

FIG. 5–18. Kielland application after clockwise rotation of right occiput transverse to occiput anterior presentation.

Posterior Presentations

Left Occiput Posterior Presentation

Assuming that the posterior fontanelle is at 4 o'clock, the blades are held in front of the patient and are locked in the position that they will occupy when applied. Therefore, the knobs point toward 4 o'clock. The anterior (right) blade is grasped, and the posterior (left) blade is temporarily discarded. The anterior blade is introduced under the symphysis to the anterior, or right, ear in the same manner as when applied to a direct transverse position. After insertion, it is rotated counterclockwise away from the occiput and toward the midline until the knob on the finger guard points toward 4 o'clock. In this instance, the rotation is made over an arc of about 135 degrees to the posterior oblique position of the head, instead of the 180-degree arc to the transverse position.

Resistance to rotation of the inverted anterior blade, which is inside the cervix, may often be overcome by carrying the handle away from the midline toward the occiput. The posterior blade is then introduced posteriorly in the oblique diameter, parallel to the sagittal suture, so that it will pass directly to the posterior ear. After the handles are locked, asynclitism is corrected by pulling down on the finger guard that is nearer to the patient's perineum while pushing up on the other finger guard. The head is then flexed and rotated counterclockwise over an arc of about 135 degrees to the anterior position. The application is checked, and traction is applied as previously described.

Right Occiput Posterior Presentation

The occiput is assumed to be at 8 o'clock in a right occiput posterior presentation. Because the right ear is posterior and the left ear is anterior, the left, or anterior, blade (the one with the lock) is introduced first. Introduction is the same as in an ROT presentation, except that, after clockwise rotation away from the occiput, the knob on the handle points to 8 o'clock instead of 9 o'clock as in the transverse position. The posterior, or right, blade is inserted posteriorly as in a left occiput posterior presentation, except that it follows the opposite oblique diameter parallel to the sagittal suture. The handles are locked, asynclitism is corrected, and the head is flexed and rotated clockwise to the anterior position. Extraction is performed in the usual manner.

Direct Occiput Posterior Presentations

The obstetrician frequently encounters situations in which the occiput engages in a posterior position or rotates posteriorly during the course of labor. If a decision is made to deliver with a forceps rotation, the Kielland forceps procedure is considered superior to the Scanzoni. A single accurate application with an instrument designed for rotation and traction is thought to be less traumatic.

With a direct occiput posterior presentation, one must be certain of the location of the fetal back in order to avoid rotation in the wrong direction. Although observation of position during labor and abdominal palpation are helpful, a quick ultrasound scan should resolve any question.

The inversion method of application is not used when the occiput is situated posteriorly and the sagittal suture points between 5 and 7 o'clock. Instead, a reverse, or upside-down, direct application is employed with the knobs facing the floor. The approach is made from below upward, with the handles at an angle of about 45 degrees below the horizontal. The operator, sitting or kneeling, applies the blades directly to the sides of the head. To facilitate locking, the right blade is always introduced first. It is inserted into the left side of the pelvis, opposite the right ear.

If the occiput is directly posterior, the forceps are held with the toes inverted and the knobs pointing downward, locked in the position of application. The right blade is taken in the left hand and introduced from below the right thigh of the patient, upward at a 45-degree angle. The toe passes directly to the right side of the fetal head, on the left side of the mother's pelvis (Figure 5–19). The left blade is then taken in the right hand and inserted from below the patient's left thigh to the left side of the head. The blades are locked, and the application is checked. If necessary, the head is flexed by elevating the handles. Rotation is accomplished by turn-

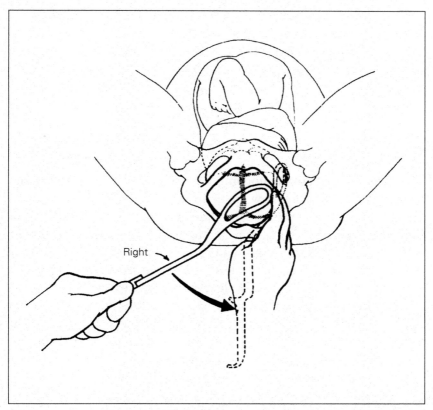

FIG. 5–19. "Upside-down direct" application of the Kielland forceps for occiput posterior presentation. The right blade, with the anterior surface of its shank pointing downward, is held in the left hand and introduced to the left side of the patient's pelvis directly to the right ear.

ing the handles through 180 degrees in the direction of the fetal back. The technique used is the same as in rotation from an occiput transverse position. The usual direction of the handles is in the midline at about 45 degrees below the horizontal, but it is higher with a lower head.

The application is similar when the occiput is found to be a few degrees away from direct occiput posterior, that is, toward 5 or 7 o'clock. The direct application is adjusted in the proper direction to maintain the blades perpendicular to the sagittal suture.

The upside-down direct application technique should not be used unless the station of the head is well down in the pelvis. If the head is at mid-station or higher, the reverse pelvic curve on the Kielland forceps interferes with application. Also, as previously noted, a fetal head at a higher station would argue against a forceps procedure. Some would consider a vacuum extractor, although abdominal delivery would probably be the procedure of choice.

Face Presentations

The use of forceps in the uncommon face presentation is somewhat limited. Most authors follow the dictum "If a face is making progress and there is no fetal heart rate abnormality, leave it alone." With greater extension of the fetal head, the biparietal diameter is higher in relation to the leading bony point. The ultimate in extension is past a brow to a face presentation. Consequently, the biparietal diameter, and thus the effective level of forceps application, is higher than the operator anticipates. Lowest-level forceps to a mentum anterior has been associated with excellent results. In other situations—namely, a higher head and transverse or posterior mentum presentations—results appear less favorable. That technique is presented for the case in which a trial at vaginal delivery appears to be indicated. The same Kielland forceps precautions, contraindications, and maneuvers apply as in previously described occiput techniques.

Anterior Chin

In face presentation with the chin anterior, a direct application to the sides of the face is made with the Kielland or a classical instrument, preferably with axis traction. Because the chin replaces the occiput as the presenting part, another exception to one of the cardinal points of forceps application arises. The left blade, instead of being applied to the left side of the face, is applied to the right side. The left blade, held in the left hand, is inserted into the left side of the vagina over the right ear. The right blade, held in the right hand, is then inserted into the right side of the vagina over the left ear. The application is checked, using the mouth as the reference point in place of the posterior fontanelle. Traction is made downward, preserving complete extension until the chin passes under the symphysis. The handles are then elevated gradually to the horizontal with traction, so that the occiput is delivered over the perineum and the head is delivered by flexion.

Transverse Chin

Rotation of a mentum transverse cannot and should not be performed unless the head is well down in the pelvis. In all face presentations, the chin takes the place of the occiput, and the Kielland forceps is applied accordingly. In a right mentum transverse presentation, the application is the same as for an ROT presentation. The left (anterior) blade is inserted first, under the symphysis to the right (anterior) ear, by the inversion method. The left blade is rotated clockwise toward the midline, away from the chin. The right blade is then inserted directly posteriorly, to the left (posterior) ear. The shanks are locked, and the chin is rotated clockwise toward 12 o'clock, bringing it under the symphysis. Downward traction is made after the application is checked. The head is delivered by flexion, following the chin under the symphysis.

In a left mentum transverse presentation, the application is the same as for an LOT presentation. Therefore, the right blade is inserted under the symphysis above the left (anterior) ear. (This is the first exception to the cardinal rule of left blade to left ear.) The toe of the blade is carried into the uterus in the inverted manner (Figure 5–20). The blade is then rotated counterclockwise away from the chin, toward the midline and toward the knob (Figure 5–21). The left blade is inserted directly posteriorly, and the shanks are locked. Counterclockwise rotation of the head brings the chin under the symphysis. Depression of the handles at the completion of rotation ensures complete extension. Traction and delivery are accomplished as in an anterior chin presentation (Figure 5–22). If the inversion method of application is thought to be inadvisable, the anterior blade may be applied by the wandering maneuver.

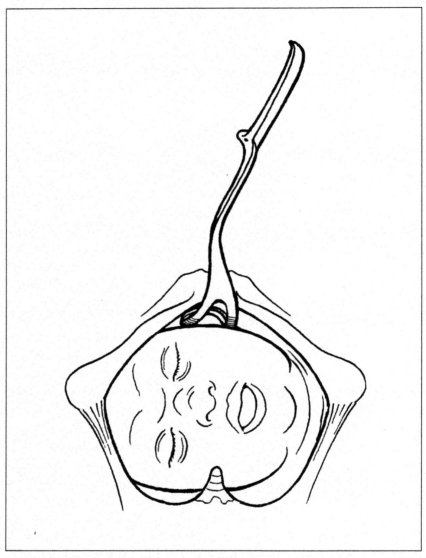

FIG. 5–20. Insertion of anterior (right) blade of Kielland forceps to anterior (left) ear of a face presentation by the inversion method in low mentum transverse presentation.

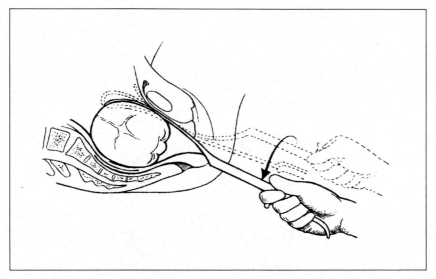

FIG. 5–21. Counterclockwise rotation of anterior (right) blade of Kielland forceps to anterior (left) ear of a face presentation in low mentum transverse presentation, so that the forceps' cephalic curve will coincide with the curve of the head.

Posterior Chin

A posterior chin presentation cannot be delivered as such with any degree of safety. If the chin is in a direct or oblique posterior position, vaginal delivery is usually not advised. The Kielland technique would be similar to that for an occiput posterior presentation, substituting the mentum as the point of reference. The head is usually at a higher level, however, and cesarean delivery is a preferable alternative.

Brow Presentation

The Kielland forceps occasionally has been used for brow presentations. When they are used, the head is either flexed or extended in order to change the brow presentation to an occiput or face presentation. Because the pivot point of the fetal head in a brow presentation is not in the center of the forceps blades, traction tends to increase extension. Also, the fetal head extension gives a higher biparietal diameter in relation to the leading bony point. Poor results attending forceps delivery of brow presentations are common, and cesarean delivery is usually preferable in these cases.

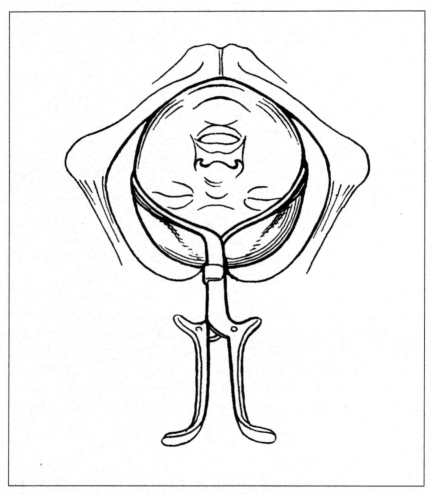

FIG. 5–22. Application of Kielland forceps to an anterior chin, ready for traction, after counterclockwise rotation of a face presentation from left mentum transverse to mentum anterior presentation.

Piper Forceps for the Aftercoming Head

The decision of whether to deliver a breech vaginally is not within the purview of this book. However, when vaginal delivery is elected, or in an emergency situation in which the breech infant is already partially delivered, the operator should consider forceps to the aftercoming head.

The use of forceps has been associated with a reduction in morbidity of up to 50% in breech deliveries. The flexion attitude of the fetal head is strictly controlled by the forceps as the head is moved through the pelvis. Because there is no traction force on the trunk or cervical spine of the infant, hyperextension injury is avoided. This is always a potential problem with other than very simple Mauriceau-Smellie-Velt maneuvers or when the head does not descend readily. Possible injury to the tentorium from suprapubic pressure on the skull is avoidable with forceps that apply force to the most resistant part, namely, the bimalar biparietal region. Delayed descent of the head subjects the infant to an increased risk of hypoxia, which is avoidable with a timely, forceps-controlled descent. The less experienced operator can be expected to lose much of the dread of vaginal breech deliveries after preparatory training and routine use of forceps to the aftercoming head.

Construction

The Piper forceps was designed in 1924 by Edmund B. Piper of Philadelphia for use on the aftercoming head in breech deliveries. The long shanks of the Piper forceps are curved backward, like a reverse pelvic curve, at about the middle. This design drops the handles to a considerable distance below the level of the blades. The other chief difference in the shanks is the development of individual planes. The plane of the shanks is the same as that of the blades to a point about 5 cm (2 inches) from the lock, whereas the lower 5 cm (2 inches) is in the plane of the handles. In the classical instrument, the plane of the shank is the same as that of the handle throughout its entire length. The unique construction of the shanks of the Piper forceps provides more spring to the blades, which in turn tends to lessen compression of the head. The blade of the Piper forceps is a modification of that of the Tarnier instrument, having a small cephalic and a slight pelvic curve.

Advantages

The dropped handles of the Piper forceps allow the instrument to be directly applied to the sides of the head without elevating the body above the horizontal, thereby preventing injury to the fetal neck. The spring of the blades, made possible because the long portion of the shanks lies in the same plane as the blades, causes less compression of the head, whereas the backward bend of the shanks provides axis traction.

Disadvantages

The blade of the Piper forceps has a straight pelvic curve and may cause some damage to the outlet during extension if an episiotomy is not performed. This is a minor consideration because the straight pelvic curve is necessary to make a direct application to a higher head. The spring in the blade, along with the slender, almost straight cephalic curve, may cause slipping on a large, round head or if the application is not accurate.

Technique

The Piper forceps should be applied after the shoulders and arms have been delivered and the head is in the pelvis with the chin posterior. The position of the head is quickly verified by feeling for the chin with the examining finger. Usually the head of a breech infant is directly posterior or within a few degrees of posterior.

An assistant is critical when a Piper forceps is used to hold the infant. The infant should be supported and the extremities removed from the field with the Savage maneuver, in which a towel sling for the infant is held by an assistant. The assistant should be cautioned against the natural impulse to improve vision by elevating the infant above the horizontal.

To avoid difficulty in locking the instrument, the left blade of the

Piper forceps is applied first. The assistant carries the infant's body toward the mother's right side, keeping it horizontal. The infant's body must never be extended over the symphysis unless the infant is "face to pubis." When the infant's body is carried toward the right side, the approach to the left side of the pelvis is more direct and less difficult.

The operator assumes a kneeling or low sitting position in front of the patient. The left blade, held in the left hand, is inserted into the left side of the pelvis over the infant's right ear (Figure 5–23). (This is the second exception to the cardinal point of left blade to left ear for forceps application.) If the head is in the anterior–posterior diameter, the left blade goes directly to the side of the pelvis. If the head is in the left occiput anterior, or right oblique diameter, the left blade is the posterior blade. When the head is in the right occiput anterior, or left oblique diameter, the left blade is the anterior blade. In each instance, the left blade is applied first, directly to the side of the head.

The handle of the forceps is held almost at right angles to the mother, below her right thigh and beneath the body of the infant, as the toe of the blade is guided into the vagina with two fingers of the operator's right hand. The handle is swept in an arc downward and toward the midline while the toe of the blade passes into the pelvis along the side of the infant's head to the right ear. The direction of the blade relative to the horizontal will vary with the station of the head but generally should be close to 45 degrees below the horizontal. Experimentation on a mannequin will show the operator that, owing to its difference from a classical instrument, the toe of the Piper forceps blade can be readily directed into the pelvic wall or sacrum if the direction is incorrect.

The assistant then carries the infant's body toward the patient's left thigh, exposing the approach to the right side of the pelvis. The right blade is similarly introduced by the right hand to the right side of the pelvis opposite the infant's left ear (Figure 5–24). If resistance is met, the toe of the blade is introduced more posteriorly and is wandered around to the side of the head. After the shanks have been locked, the infant is allowed to straddle the forceps. The handles rest

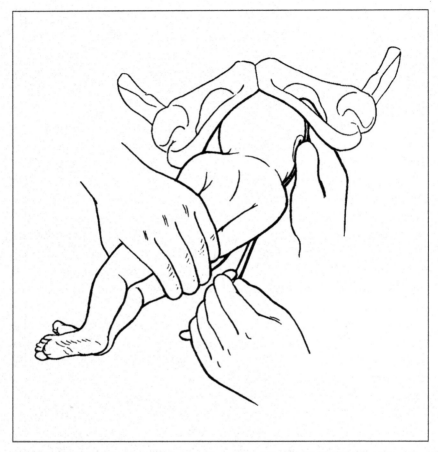

FIG. 5–23. Insertion, from below and upward, of first (left) blade of the Piper forceps to the right ear of the aftercoming head.

in the upturned palm of the operator's right hand with the middle finger in the space between the shanks.

After application of the forceps, if the head is not in a direct anterior position, it is rotated instrumentally and downward traction is made from the kneeling or sitting position in the direction of the handles until the chin appears at the outlet. The handles are then elevated with traction in order to conform to the curve of the pelvis and to promote and preserve flexion during delivery of the head over the perineum. As traction is made, the right thumb grasps the

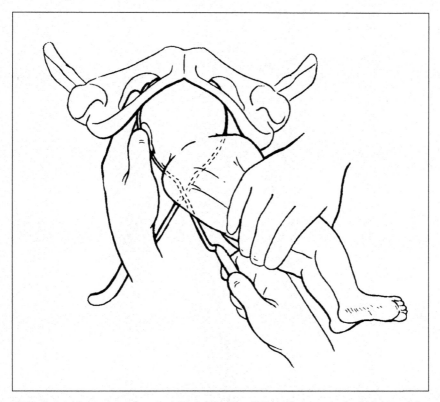

FIG. 5–24. Insertion of second (right) blade of Piper forceps to the left ear of the aftercoming head.

infant's thigh over the forceps handles, so that when the head is extracted it will not fall through the blades. The index and middle fingers of the operator's left hand press on the suboccipital region, splinting the neck and helping to bring the occiput under the arch (Figure 5–25). If resistance is encountered at the outlet after an episiotomy has been performed, the handles of the blades are depressed and elevated during gentle traction in a pump-handle maneuver. This favors delivery of the head over the perineum with less effort and less injury; first, by bringing the suboccipital region further under the arch, and second, by increasing the flexion. Finally, extraction is performed with the handles close to the horizontal, delivering the head with the forceps still in place (Figure 5–26).

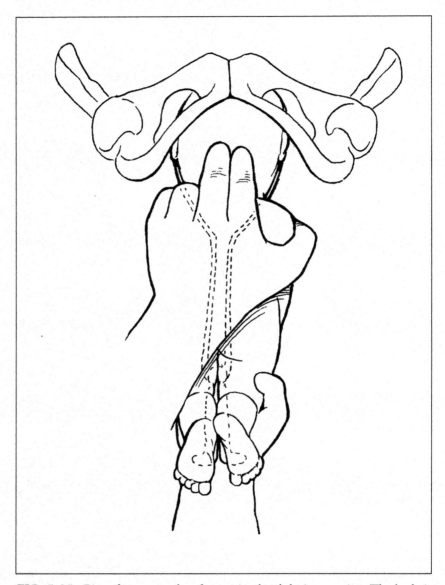

FIG. 5–25. Piper forceps on the aftercoming head during traction. The body is resting on the shanks of the forceps, the leg is clamped to the handle by the operator's thumb, the handles are resting in the upturned palm of the operator's right hand with the middle finger in the space between the shanks at the lock, and the neck is splinted by the fingers of the operator's left hand.

The very rare "face-to-pubis" situation is usually avoided by the method of delivery of the body, shoulders, and arms. If a face-up aftercoming head is encountered, the forceps are applied if a bimanual maneuver fails to deliver the aftercoming head. The approach is made from below upward, under the infant's back, directly to the sides of the head, the leading point of which is now the occiput. After traction is applied, the occiput is delivered over the perineum with the chin facing the pubis. Simultaneously, the legs and body are carried up over the symphysis.

A classical type of forceps may be used on the aftercoming head, but its disadvantages make this rather undesirable. The pelvic curve and the straight shanks of the classical type of forceps require elevation of the infant's body toward the symphysis to permit application of the blades beneath it. This risks injury to the neck and tends to extend the head. Moreover, the forward bend of the shanks and handles tends to interfere with complete instrumental flexion of the head. The rigid blades can give more compression to the head. Unless the instrument has such an attachment, axis traction cannot be utilized.

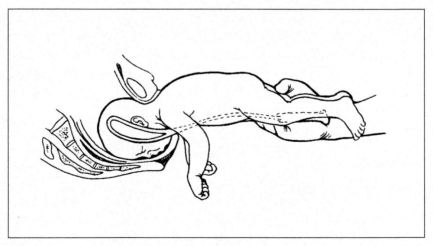

FIG. 5–26. Application of Piper forceps to the aftercoming head, which is about to be delivered over the perineum by flexion without removal of the forceps.

Bill Handle

Special instruments that apply the axis traction principle are available. The importance of axis traction cannot be underestimated. As previously stated, to use the least force in accomplishing descent of the head, traction must be in the pelvic axis. Manual methods of axis traction, at any level of the pelvis, require an estimation of the relative forces being applied. This is essentially the obstetrician's subjective impression and carries the potential for deviation from the optimal course. The possibility of trauma to fetus and mother is lessened by an instrument or attachment that decreases force wasted in the wrong direction. In addition, the operator can more easily evaluate the amount of traction force actually applied to the head when the vectored force is supplied by an axis traction instrument and is a straight pull.

The Bill axis traction handle is an important addition to the range of available instruments in that it is a device that attaches to a classical instrument, resulting in automatic axis traction (Figure 5–27). The Bill handle has two shafts connected with a hinge. At the hinge is a lateral marker that indicates the correct position of the hinge when in use. One shaft ends in hooks that slip over the linger guards of the previously applied forceps. The other shaft ends in the traction bar, which is dropped over the perineum, down into the long axis of the head. No vectoring of forces is necessary because tractive force on the handle is directly applied in the proper direction (assuming correct application has been performed). This greatly facilitates traction.

Vectis

One blade of a forceps or a special instrument may be used as a vectis to assist in delivery of the head through the uterine incision during cesarean delivery. The operator's hand, cupped beneath the head and aiding extraction, greatly increases the necessary circumference of the uterine incision. Extensions of the incision are

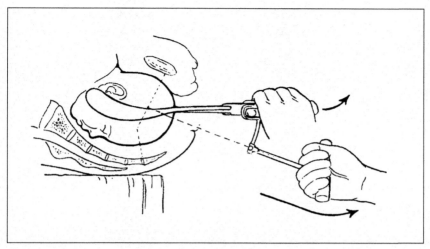

FIG. 5–27. Instrumental axis traction. Tucker-McLane forceps, solid blades with Bill handle.

not uncommon, may be difficult to repair, and involve extra blood loss.

A vectis aids rotation and elevation of the head and helps to deliver the head by extension, as in vaginal delivery. It can act similarly to an inclined plane, directing the head when fundal pressure is applied. It occupies very little space, and extensions of the incision are rarely needed.

Although a single forceps blade may be used, the type of vectis that is symmetrical, having only a fenestrated cephalic curve on a shank and handle, is easier to use. The operator inserts one hand in the uterine incision, feeling the direction of the sagittal suture, as the toe of the vectis is inserted. The vectis is then moved between the operator's fingers and the infant's head, usually over the parietal bone. The operator's hand is removed and the vectis is lifted and turned to direct the occiput upward and through the incision, propelled by fundal pressure.

The use of a special, short Simpson-type forceps, and even the vacuum extractor, have also been advocated for extraction of the head during cesarean delivery. These instruments are felt to be more cumbersome and time consuming. It is always advisable to deliver the fetal head in as short a time as possible after the uterine incision has been made.

CHAPTER 6

Posterior Presentations of the Occiput

*P*osterior presentations are managed either by manual or instrumental rotation to the anterior position, or by a combination of these two methods, when there are maternal or fetal indications for delivery. Special instruments (see Chapter 5) may be used for this purpose. Less frequently, certain situations are met in which delivery should be performed as an occiput posterior (OP) presentation.

Manual Rotation: Left and Right Occiput Posterior Presentations

Manual rotation of a posterior head is accomplished in the same manner as for a transverse head, with the exception that the head must be rotated over a longer arc to the anterior position. The operator's right hand is the rotating hand for a left occiput posterior (LOP) presentation (Figure 6–1), and the left hand is the rotating hand for a right occiput posterior (ROP) presentation. After manual rotation to an anterior quadrant of the pelvis has been accomplished, the thumb of the rotating hand is removed from the vagina while pressure is placed on the fundus by an assistant. The four fingers remain in place behind the posterior parietal bone to splint the head and prevent it from rotating back to the transverse or posterior position while the posterior blade is being applied. The blade in left-sided positions of the occiput is the left blade. Its handle is held in the left hand, and it is inserted into the left side of the

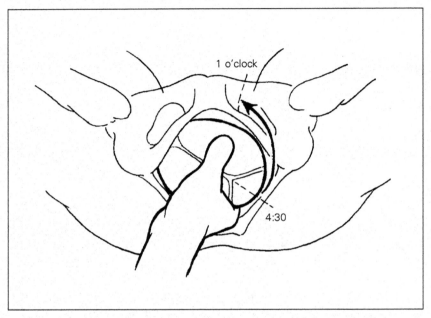

FIG. 6–1. Manual rotation of left occiput posterior to anterior presentation with the operator's right hand.

pelvis opposite the left ear. In right-sided positions, it is the right blade, held with the handle in the right hand. After the posterior blade has been placed in position opposite the posterior ear, the fingers of the rotating hand are removed from the vagina so that they can hold the handle of the anterior blade. This is introduced in the usual manner for an anterior position. The shanks then are locked, the application is checked, and rotation to occiput anterior (OA) is completed. The application is rechecked, and any necessary readjustments are made before extraction is begun.

Combined Manual and Instrumental Rotation

If manual rotation of a posterior head cannot be accomplished beyond the transverse position, it may be completed instrumentally by applying the forceps as in a transverse arrest. The rotating hand is kept in place to act as a splint while the posterior blade is being applied (Figure 6–2). The anterior blade is wandered around the brow by the elevating fingers at the heel as the handle is depressed well below the handle of the posterior blade. When the blade is in place behind the symphysis opposite the anterior ear, the handle is elevated to the locking position beneath the handle of the posterior blade. Instrumental rotation of the head to the OA position is completed in a counterclockwise direction for left-sided positions. In right-sided positions, the direction of rotation is clockwise. After the application is checked, traction is applied.

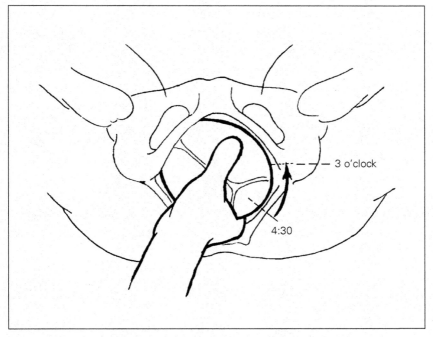

FIG. 6–2. Manual rotation of left occiput posterior to left occiput transverse presentation preparatory to application of Elliot forceps to left occiput transverse presentation, using the wandering method for the anterior blade and completion of rotation to occiput anterior presentation instrumentally.

Instrumental Rotation: Modified Scanzoni Maneuver in Left Occiput Posterior Presentation

The modified Scanzoni maneuver consists of complete instrumental rotation, with an Elliot type of forceps, of an occiput posterior presentation to the anterior position. This is accomplished with a single maneuver, but a reapplication of the forceps is required for completion of the delivery.

An LOP presentation is considered as a right occiput anterior presentation, and the blades are applied accordingly. In an LOP presentation, the right blade is held in the right hand and is applied first, into the right side of the pelvis and over the left (posterior) ear (Figure 6–3). (This is the third exception to the cardinal point of the right blade to the right ear.) After the right blade is applied, the left blade is taken in the left hand and applied to the left side of the pelvis to the right, or anterior, ear. The handles are crossed and the shanks locked (Figure 6–4). A preliminary check should show the posterior fontanelle to be just below the plane of the shanks and the sagittal suture perpendicular to the plane of the shanks. The head is then rotated counterclockwise to the anterior position. The pelvic curve of the forceps makes it necessary to rotate the handles over a wide arc to keep the blades in the center of the pelvis, thereby avoiding obstruction or injury. Frequently, the head is extended, resulting in a deviation of the long axis of the head from the axis of the pelvis. If flexion is performed first, rotation will be made much easier because resistance will be decreased. If the widest part of the head is arrested at the plane of the ischial spines, it will be necessary to push it up 1–2 cm to bring it close to the plane of greatest pelvic dimension before rotation. Rotation at the inlet is not advised.

In LOP positions, rotation is counterclockwise. After the handles are elevated in order to produce flexion, and after they are rotated in order to bring the occiput into the anterior oblique (left occiput anterior [LOA]) diameter of the pelvis, the head is fixed in the new position by slight downward traction. Because the blades are now upside-down, with the toes pointing posteriorly, they must be removed, inverted, and reapplied (Figure 6–5). The posterior (right)

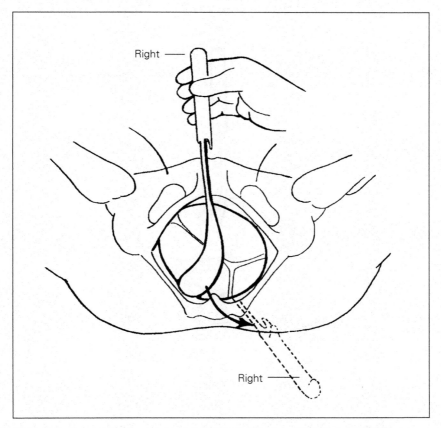

FIG. 6–3. Insertion of posterior (right) blade (Tucker–McLane), solid Elliot type, in the first stage of the modified Scanzoni maneuver for instrumental rotation of left occiput posterior to occiput anterior presentation.

blade, which is the one over the left ear, is temporarily retained in place to splint the head in the anterior position. The anterior blade is removed first, in a downward direction (Figure 6–6). Because it is the left blade, it is reinserted between the head and the blade that is still in place opposite the left ear, as in the LOA technique (Figure 6–7). After this is accomplished, the right, or "splinting," blade is removed in a downward direction and reapplied over the right, or anterior, ear (Figure 6–8). In the original Scanzoni maneuver, first introduced in the 19th century, both blades are removed after the

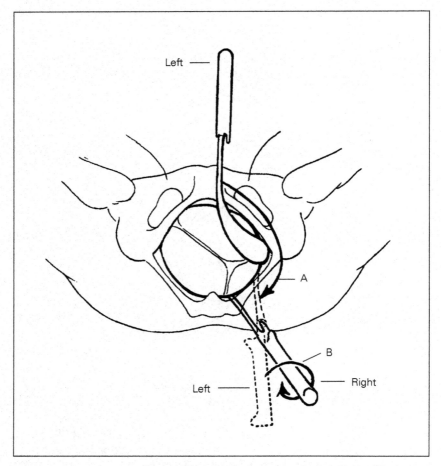

FIG. 6–4. Insertion of anterior (left) blade and crossing the handle, left over right, for locking in the first stage of the modified Scanzoni maneuver for left occiput posterior presentation.

head is rotated to the anterior quadrant of the pelvis, and the posterior blade is not left in place as a splint. The blades are then reapplied to the new anterior position. Frequently, the head rotates back toward the original position before reapplication can be made. The modified Scanzoni maneuver is preferable to the original maneuver in that the head is less likely to slip back to the transverse or posterior position due to the presence of the splinting blade.

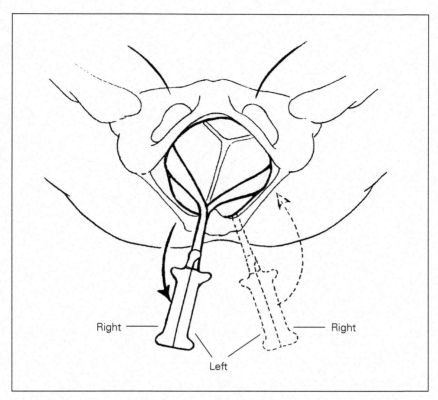

FIG. 6–5. Instrumental rotation counterclockwise from left occiput posterior to anterior presentation. This completes the first stage of the modified Scanzoni maneuver. The occiput is now anterior, but the blades are upside-down. The second stage involves removal, reinversion, and reapplication.

In performing this modified Scanzoni maneuver, it has been found that the Elliot type of forceps with overlapping shanks, especially the solid-bladed Tucker-McLane, or the Luikart modification, is preferable because it offers less resistance to application, rotation, and removal. In addition, the Bill axis traction handle can be used as an aid to rotation as well as traction. If desired, a different type of instrument with a fenestrated blade may be used for the second application and for traction. It is very easy to slip a fenestrated blade between the head and a solid posterior splinting blade. Using a solid blade for rotation obviates the possibility of threading

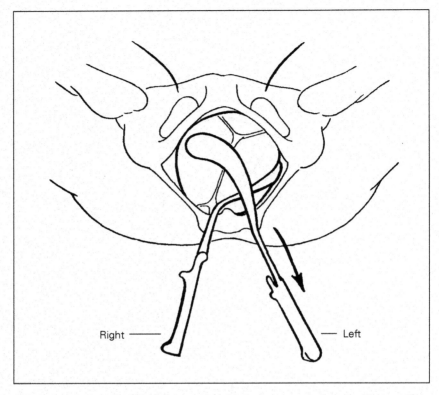

Right —————   ————— Left

FIG. 6–6. Removal of the left (anterior) blade downward after one fixing pull in this direction.

the reapplied blade through the fenestration of the splinting blade. Should this happen, it complicates the removal of the splinting blade. In this case, removal can be facilitated by withdrawing the blade along the surrounded shank, past the finger guard, to the end of the handle.

It must be emphasized that, after rotation of the head to the anterior position in the first stage of this maneuver, the blades are upside-down, so that the pelvic curve is facing the sacrum. Therefore, removal of the blades must be accomplished by pulling downward on the handles toward the floor. After the head has been rotated to the OA position, the reapplication is checked, and if it is found to be satisfactory, traction is begun (Figure 6–9).

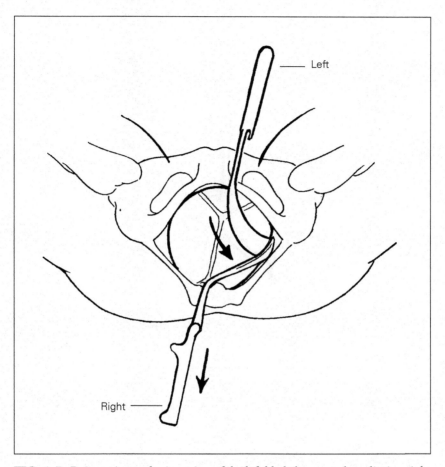

FIG. 6–7. Reinversion and reinsertion of the left blade between the splinting right blade and the posterior (left) ear, as for left occiput anterior presentation.

Scanzoni Maneuver in Right Occiput Posterior Presentation

To perform the Scanzoni maneuver in an ROP presentation, the ROP position is considered as an LOA. The blades are applied, and the head is rotated clockwise to the anterior quadrant. Removal and reapplication are similar to that used in an LOP presentation, except that in the second application (ie, to the new right occiput

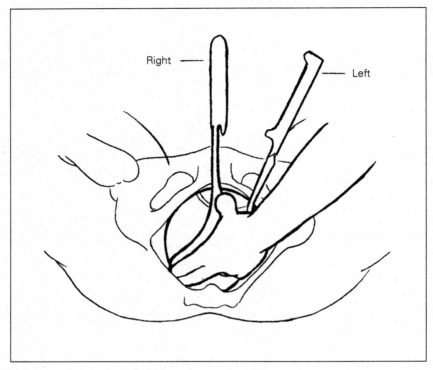

FIG. 6–8. Reapplication of the right splinting blade to the anterior (right) ear as in left occiput anterior presentation, after removal in a downward direction and reinversion.

anterior position), the handles must be crossed in order to lock them prior to traction.

Directly Posterior Heads (Occiput Posterior Presentations)

The occiput in the direct posterior position is treated similarly to one in the transverse or posterior oblique position, except that it is rotated over a longer arc to the anterior position. The rotation may be performed manually or instrumentally. Before attempting the rotation, it is necessary to know on which side the fetal back lies in

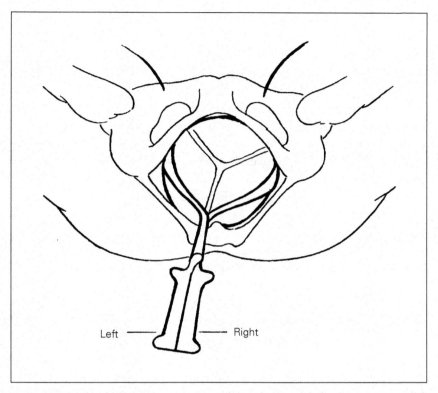

FIG. 6–9. The forceps are now properly applied and locked in the new left occiput anterior position, ready for traction after completing rotation to occiput anterior position. The Bill handle should be added for traction.

order to determine which way to rotate the head. This avoids the danger of injury to the neck from rotation in the wrong direction. The occiput should rotate through the side on which the back lies. Because a fetal position with the back posterior is rare, the back can be identified by abdominal palpation or ultrasound scan. If the back is to the left, the rotation is counterclockwise, using the same technique as in an LOP presentation. If the back is on the right side, rotation is clockwise as in an ROP presentation. After rotation has been accomplished, forceps application (or reapplication, if a Scanzoni maneuver is being used) and traction are performed as previously described.

The DeLee "key-in-lock" maneuver is a gradual instrumental rotation of an occiput posterior to the anterior position by multiple readjustments of the forceps. This is accomplished with application as though the posterior occiput were anterior. The instrument, classically a DeLee–Simpson forceps, rotates the head through a 15–20-degree arc in the proper direction. It is then unlocked and readjusted, and the movement is repeated. The head is rotated in steps through 180 degrees as the instrument remains in the anterior quadrants. This maneuver has been popular in some areas but generally has been supplanted by methods that avoid asymmetrical stress to the fetal skull. It is presented here as mainly of historic interest.

Delivery as an Occiput Posterior Presentation

Occasionally, in an anthropoid pelvis with a transverse diameter that is too narrow to permit anterior rotation, a posterior occiput presentation should be delivered as such. The same procedure is used in a case of a marked "funnel" pelvis, usually android, with the occiput posterior head molded into the outlet under a narrow arch.

For several reasons, delivery as a posterior is not a simple one. More force is required to accomplish descent of the occiput posterior head. Because the head is being moved in an awkward direction that is opposite to normal, the direction of the traction force is critical to avoid trauma to the head. With extension and molding of the head, the biparietal diameter may be at a higher level than anticipated. Considerably more soft tissue space is required, and the risk for a fourth-degree episiotomy extension is much greater. In our opinion, this should not be classified as an outlet forceps procedure, regardless of the station of the head.

An instrument employing the axis traction principle is preferred. The technique of application of forceps to an occiput posterior presentation that is to be delivered without anterior rotation is similar to that for the first stage of the Scanzoni maneuver Before the handles are locked, they are depressed against the perineum until the shanks are close to the level of the posterior fontanelle. More effort in traction is necessary for delivery of an occiput posterior presentation as such. After the anterior fontanelle appears under the symphysis, the head is delivered by flexion instead of by extension.

This discussion of posterior and transverse heads deals only with the use of the classical instruments. Many cases are handled more efficiently with less manipulation and less effort if the operator uses a special instrument, such as the Kielland forceps. Certain modifications of classical instruments may also be used to manage posterior heads. The operative management of occiput posterior positions is shown in the box.

Operative Management of Occiput Posterior Positions

1. Manual rotation to occiput anterior
   A. Digital rotation } Followed by Simpson type;
   B. Manual rotation } best with axis traction

2. Combined manual and instrumental rotation to occiput anterior
   Wandering maneuver, Elliot-type forceps, after manual or digital rotation to transverse

3. Instrumental rotation to occiput anterior
   A. Classical instruments
      (a) Scanzoni maneuver (modified)
          Elliot-type forceps (solid blade: Tucker-McLane, Luikart)
      (b) DeLee "key in lock" maneuver (not recommended), Simpson-type forceps
   B. Modified classical instruments: Jacobs–Elliot type, solid blade
   C. Special instruments: Kielland

4. Deliver as a posterior position
   A. Android pelvis—selected cases (Simpson type, axis traction)
   B. Anthropoid pelvis—selected cases (Simpson type, axis traction)

Note: Internal podalic version, listed in the past as an alternative, is no longer considered to be acceptable.

Chapter 7

Vacuum Assisted Delivery*

lthough the principle of suction has been used in medicine for many years, its application to obstetrics did not become popularized until Malström reported his experience in 1954 (1). His original instrument used a steel cup that was attached to a chain for traction. This chain was threaded through the suction hose and suction was applied by use of a suction pump. The original caps were designed to create a caput that was smaller at the base and expanded within the cup. The caps were 40, 50, and 60 mm in size. Since this early introduction, there have been a number of modifications designed to make the vacuum easier to use. In 1969, Bird reported on a modification that removed the chain from inside the hose and attached it to the outside of the cup for ease in traction (2). In the late 1970s and early 1980s, there were experiments with replacing the metal cups with Silastic plastic cups. Originally, these cups were cone-shaped with built-in handles. Subsequent modifications have altered their appearance so they more closely reflect their metal counterparts. In 1985, Berkus reported on a cohort study with use of the Silastic cup indicating its effectiveness and safety (3). Further refinements have also included a hand pump rather than an electric pump and modifications in the structure. Today, the vacuum extractor has achieved a position similar to that of forceps in the obstetric management of patients.

---

*Adapted from American College of Obstetricians and Gynecologists. Operative Vaginal Delivery. ACOG Practice Bulletin 17. Washington, DC: ACOG, 2000

Technique

The application of the cup should be applied in the same clinical situations where forceps are considered. It is critical that there be complete cervical dilatation because parts of the cervix, if present, can be pulled into the cup. The largest size of cup that can be easily positioned over the vertex should be used. A critical aspect of application is to proceed slowly in raising the caput. The negative pressure should not exceed 0.6 to 0.8 kg/cm^2 of pressure. This is obtained by using an initial vacuum of 0.2 kg/cm^2 to hold the cup in place. Then every 2 minutes an additional 0.2 kg/cm^2 should be applied until the maximum is reached.

Traction should only be applied once the maximum negative pressure has been attained. The preferred method is to apply traction during the patient's uterine contraction and resting during the interval between contractions. As with forceps, traction should attempt to follow the pelvic curvature. If necessary, the cup can be gently rotated during traction by the free hand. Care should be taken to allow the woman's pushing and the fetal descent to assist in the rotation rather than attempting an unassisted rotation as occurs with forceps.

The delivery should be completed within 30 minutes or the cup should be removed. Longer applications can result in injury to the scalp. Deliveries generally occur within five pulls although this is variable. The most valuable index is whether the fetal head is descending or remaining stationary. If the latter, the potential for cephalopelvic disproportion must be evaluated. Occasionally the cup will be pulled from the scalp. This usually does not occur but when it does the physician needs to reevaluate the vacuum application, the traction force and direction. If these are correct and the cup pulls free a second time, it may be preferable to consider a cesarean delivery.

Potential Complications to the Infant

Vacuum extractors are designed to limit the amount of traction on the fetal skull because detachment can occur. Nevertheless, traction achieved with vacuum extraction is substantial (up to 50 lb) (4) and can result in significant fetal injury if misused.

The incidence of subgaleal hematomas (collections of blood occurring in the potential space between the cranial periosteum and the epicranial aponeurosis) following vacuum deliveries is estimated to range from 26 to 45 per 1,000 vacuum deliveries (5, 6). Other potential neonatal complications associated with vacuum deliveries include intracranial hemorrhage, hyperbilirubinemia, and retinal hemorrhage. The higher rates of neonatal jaundice associated with vacuum delivery may be related to the higher rate of cephalohematoma (7). There is a higher rate of retinal hemorrhages (38%) with vacuum delivery than with forceps delivery (17%) (8–11). However, corneal abrasions and external ocular trauma are more common with forceps delivery than with normal spontaneous delivery and are rare with vacuum extraction unless the cup is inadvertently placed over the eye. Long-term sequelae are extremely rare, and ophthalmologic screening should be reserved for specific cases (11). Overall, the incidence of serious complications with vacuum extraction is approximately 5% (12).

In 1998, the U.S. Food and Drug Administration (FDA) released a Public Health Advisory to alert individuals that vacuum extractors may cause serious or fatal complications, including subgaleal (subaponeurotic) hematoma and intracranial hemorrhage (13). The FDA indicated that between 1994 and 1998, 12 deaths and nine serious injuries were reported among neonates on whom vacuum-assisted devices had been used. This rate was greater than five times the rate for the preceding 11 years. According to the advisory, data collected from 1989 to 1995 showed that use of the vacuum cup had increased from 3.5% to 5.9% of all deliveries. Among the FDA recommendations for use of the vacuum device, two are particularly useful:

1. Rocking movements or torque should not be applied to the device; only steady traction in the line of the birth canal should be used.
2. Clinicians caring for the neonate should be alerted that a vacuum device has been used so that they can adequately monitor the neonate for the signs and symptoms of device-related injuries.

A recent study evaluating the incidence of severe birth trauma following operative deliveries assessed the outcome of 83,340 singleton infants born to nulliparous women between 1992 and 1994 in California (14). A database was created linking birth and death certificates with hospital discharge records of maternal and neonatal outcomes. The lowest risk of fetal injury was found in infants delivered spontaneously. An intermediate risk was observed for those infants delivered by forceps or vacuum alone or by cesarean delivery during labor. The highest risk of fetal injury was reported for those infants who were delivered with combined forceps and vacuum extraction or who were delivered by cesarean following failed operative vaginal delivery. There was no difference in outcome between vacuum and forceps delivery versus cesarean delivery during labor (Table 1). The morbidity that previously had been thought to be due to operative vaginal delivery actually may have resulted from the process of abnormal labor that led to the need for intervention. The study population was large, but data were collected retrospectively from medical records and hospital discharge

TABLE 1. Effect of Delivery on Neonatal Injury

Delivery Method	Death	Intracranial Hemorrhage	Other*
Spontaneous vaginal delivery	1/5,000	1/1,900	1/216
Cesarean delivery during labor	1/1,250	1/952	1/71
Cesarean delivery after vacuum/forceps	N/R	1/333	1/38
Cesarean delivery with no labor	1/1,250	1/2,040	1/105
Vacuum alone	1/3,333	1/860	1/122
Forceps alone	1/2,000	1/664	1/76
Vacuum and forceps	1/1,666	1/280	1/58

Abbreviation: N/R indicates not reported.

*Facial nerve/brachial plexus injury, convulsions, central nervous system depression, mechanical ventilation

Data from Towner D, Castro MA, Eby-Wilkens E, Gilbert WM. Effect of mode of delivery in nulliparous women on neonatal intracranial injury. N Engl J Med 1999;341:1709–1714 reports. Therefore, detailed information on the operative vaginal delivery, frequency of congenital anomalies, or number of infants readmitted following the initial discharge was not available.

One randomized comparison of vacuum versus forceps delivery that evaluated children at 9 months of age found no statistically significant differences between the two groups regarding head circumference, weight, head-circumference-to-weight ratio, hearing, or vision (15). The study did note that infants delivered with the vacuum device were more likely to have been readmitted with jaundice than were those delivered with forceps.

A 10-year matched follow-up evaluation of 295 children delivered by vacuum extractor and 302 control patients who had been delivered spontaneously at the same hospital revealed no differences between the two groups in terms of scholastic performance, speech, ability of self-care, or neurologic abnormality (16).

One study showed that in cases in which the vacuum extractor was used to deliver fetuses with nonreassuring fetal heart rate patterns, blood gas parameters did not differ from those in cases with normal spontaneous deliveries. The authors concluded that the use of vacuum extraction is not contraindicated in cases of nonreassuring fetal heart rate patterns (17).

Potential Maternal Complications

A larger randomized study comparing outlet forceps delivery with spontaneous vaginal delivery in 333 women at term showed that, although the use of forceps had no immediate adverse effects on the neonate, there was no significant shortening of the second stage of labor. However, the incidence of maternal perineal trauma increased in primiparous women (18).

A meta-analysis comparing vacuum extraction to forceps delivery showed that vacuum extraction was associated with significantly less maternal trauma and less need for general and regional anesthesia. Overall, fewer cesarean deliveries were carried out in the vacuum extractor group (8). Other studies comparing vacuum extraction to forceps delivery indicate that more maternal morbidity (soft tissue injury, discomfort) occurs with forceps delivery (9, 19). A randomized study of forceps and vacuum-assisted vaginal delivery identified three factors associated with the development of shoulder dystocia: use of vacuum device ($P = 0.04$), time required for delivery ($P = 0.03$), and birth weight ($P = 0.0001$) (20).

Special Circumstances

Occasionally an operator will have a failure with the vacuum and wish to resort to forceps. A California study reported that the incidence of intracranial hemorrhage was highest in infants delivered by combined vacuum and forceps compared with other reported methods of delivery (14). The incidences of other injuries also were increased with combined methods of operative vaginal delivery.

Randomized trials comparing soft vacuum cups to the original metal cup indicate that the pliable cup is associated with decreased fetal scalp trauma but increased rates of detachment from the fetal head (21–24). However, there are no differences between Apgar scores, cord pH, neurologic outcome, retinal hemorrhage, maternal trauma, and blood loss (24). These findings support those of another study, which found a 22% incidence of significant fetal scalp trauma with the soft cup, as opposed to a 37% incidence with the metal cup. This study also concluded the soft cup was more likely to fail than the metal cup when excessive caput was present (21).

Data show that the use of rapid vacuum application leads to a reduction in time to delivery (25, 26). No differences in detachment from the fetal scalp or in maternal or neonatal morbidity between the two techniques have been noted (25, 26). Specifically, one randomized study of 94 women comparing a one-step rapid application of vacuum with conventional stepwise application of vacuum found a significant reduction in the time from application to delivery (6 minutes) in the rapid application group without any differences in maternal or neonatal morbidity (25).

Cephalohematoma has been shown to be more likely to develop as the duration of vacuum application increases. One study demonstrated that 28% of neonates in whom the application-to-delivery time exceeded 5 minutes developed cephalohematoma (27).

A randomized controlled trial involving 322 patients at 34 weeks or more of gestation highlighted factors involved in the development of fetal cephalohematoma from vacuum extraction using the M-cup (a semirigid plastic cup, modeled after the Malmstrom cup). To prevent fetal loss of station, 164 patients had continuous vacuum application (600 mm Hg) during and between contractions as well as during active efforts at delivery. In the comparison group, 158 patients had intermittent suction (reduction of vacuum application to 100 mm Hg between contractions) and no effort to prevent loss of station between contractions. Time to delivery, method failure, maternal lacerations, episiotomy extension, incidence of cephalohematoma, and neonatal outcome were similar between the two groups. Overall, the efficacy of the vacuum cup was 93.5%, and the cephalohematoma rate was 11.5%. The authors concluded that there are no differences in maternal or fetal outcome with intermittent reduction in vacuum or attempts to prevent loss of station. They also concluded that the results obtained with the M-cup are comparable to those reported with the stainless-steel Malmstrom cup (28).

Summary

Both forceps and vacuum extractors are acceptable and safe instruments for operative vaginal delivery. Operator experience should determine which instrument should be used in a particular situation.

The vacuum extractor is associated with an increased incidence of neonatal cephalohematomata, retinal hemorrhages, and jaundice when compared with forceps delivery. Operators should attempt to minimize the duration of vacuum application, because cephalohematoma is more likely to occur as the interval increases.

Midforceps operations should be considered an appropriate procedure to teach and to use under the correct circumstances by an adequately trained individual. The incidence of intracranial hemorrhage is highest among infants delivered by cesarean following a failed vacuum or forceps delivery. The combination of vacuum and forceps has a similar incidence of intracranial hemorrhage. Therefore, an operative vaginal delivery should not be attempted when the probability of success is very low.

References

1. Malström T. Vacuum extractor: an obstetrical instrument. Acta Obstet Gynecol Scand 1954;33 (suppl 4)

2. Modifications of Malstrom's vacuum extractor. Br Med J 1969;3:526

3. Berkus MD, Ramamurthy RS, O'Connor PS, Brown K, Hayashi RH. Cohort study of silastic obstetric vacuum cup deliveries: I. Safety of the instrument. Obstet Gynecol 1985;66:503–509

4. Moolgaoker AS, Ahamed SOS, Payne PR. A comparison of different methods of instrumental delivery based on electronic measurements of compression and traction. Obstet Gynecol 1979;54:299–309

5. Boo NY. Subaponeurotic haemorrhage in Malaysian neonates. Singapore Med J 1990;31:207–210

6. Govaert P, Defoort P, Wigglesworth JS. Cranial haemorrhage in the term newborn infant. Clin Dev Med 1993;129:1–223

7. Vacca A, Grant A, Wyatt G, Chalmers I. Portsmouth operative delivery trial: a comparison of vacuum extraction and forceps delivery. Br J Obstet Gynaecol 1983;90: 1107–1112

8. Johanson RB, Menon BKV. Vacuum extraction versus forceps for assisted vaginal delivery (Cochrane Review). In: The Cochrane Library, Issue 4, 1999. Oxford: Update Software

9. Dell DL, Sightler SE, Plauche WC. Soft cup vacuum extraction: a comparison of outlet delivery. Obstet Gynecol 1985;66:624–628

10. Williams MC, Knuppel RA, O'Brien WF, Weiss A, Kanarek KS. A randomized comparison of assisted vaginal delivery by obstetric forceps and polyethylene vacuum cup. Obstet Gynecol 1991; 78:789–794

11. Holden R, Morsman DG, Davidek GM, O'Connor GM, Coles EC, Dawson AJ. External ocular trauma in instrumental and normal deliveries. Br J Obstet Gynaecol 1992;99:132–134

12. Robertson PA, Laros RK Jr, Zhao RL. Neonatal and maternal outcome in low-pelvic and midpelvic operative deliveries. Am J Obstet Gynecol 1990;162:1436–1442; discussion 1442–1444

13. Center for Devices and Radiological Health. FDA Public Health Advisory: need for caution when using vacuum assisted delivery devices. May 21, 1998. Available at http://www.fda.gov/cdrh/fetal598.html. Retrieved December 31, 1999

14. Towner D, Castro MA, Eby-Wilkens E, Gilbert WM. Effect of mode of delivery in nulliparous women on neonatal intracranial injury. N Engl J Med 1999; 341:1709–1714

15. Carmody F, Grant A, Mutch L, Vacca A, Chalmers I. Follow up of babies delivered in a randomized controlled comparison of vacuum extraction and forceps delivery. Acta Obstet Gynecol Scand 1986;65:763–766

16. Ngan HY, Miu P, Ko L, Ma HK. Long-term neurological sequelae following vacuum extractor delivery. Aust N Z J Obstet Gynaecol 1990;30:111–114

17. Vintzileos AM, Nochimson DJ, Antsaklis A, Varvarigos I, Guzman ER, Knuppel RA. Effect of vacuum extraction on umbilical cord blood acid-base measurements. J Matern Fetal Med 1996;5:11–17

18. Yancey MK, Herpolsheimer A, Jordan GD, Benson WL, Brady K. Maternal and neonatal effects of outlet forceps delivery compared with spontaneous vaginal delivery in term pregnancies. Obstet Gynecol 1991;78:646–650

19. Johanson R, Pusey J, Livera N, Jones P. North Staffordshire/Wigan assisted delivery trial. Br J Obstet Gynaecol 1989;96:537–544

20. Bofill JA, Rust OA, Devidas M, Roberts WE, Morrison JC, Martin JN Jr. Shoulder dystocia and operative vaginal delivery. J Matern Fetal Med 1997;6:220–224

21. Chenoy R, Johanson R. A randomized prospective study comparing delivery with metal and silicone rubber vacuum extractor cups. Br J Obstet Gynaecol 1992;99:360–363

22. Cohn M, Barclay C, Fraser R, Zaklama M, Johanson R, Anderson D, et al. A mulitcentre randomized trial comparing delivery with a silicone rubber cup and rigid metal vacuum extractor cups. Br J Obstet Gynaecol 1989;96: 545–551

23. Hofmeyr GJ, Gobetz L, Sonnendecker EW, Turner MJ. New design rigid and soft vacuum extractor cups: a preliminary comparison of traction forces. Br J Obstet Gynaecol 1990;97:681–685

24. Kuit JA, Eppinga HG, Wallenburg HC, Huikeshoven FJ. A randomized comparison of vacuum extraction delivery with a rigid and a pliable cup. Obstet Gynecol 1993; 82:280–284

25. Lim FT, Holm JP, Schuitemaker NW, Jansen FH, Hermans J. Stepwise compared with rapid application of vacuum in ventouse extraction procedures. Br J Obstet Gynaecol 1997;104:33–36

26. Svenningsen L. Birth progression and traction forces developed under vacuum extraction after slow or rapid application of suction. Eur J Obstet Gynecol Reprod Biol 1987;26:105–112

27. Bofill JA, Rust OA, Devidas M, Roberts WE, Morrison JC, Martin JN Jr. Neonatal cephalohematoma from vacuum extraction. J Reprod Med 1997;42:565–569

28. Bofill JA, Rust OA, Schorr SJ, Brown RC, Roberts WE, Morrison JC. A randomized trial of two vacuum extraction techniques. Obstet Gynecol 1997;89:758–762

CHAPTER 8

Special Considerations

*M*any choices arise when the obstetrician is presented with a situation in which there is a fetal or maternal indication for intervention with the course of a labor. The variables in a clinical situation are essentially limitless. They must be evaluated, however, in an effort to decide the most appropriate action within the given circumstances.

All of the prerequisites for forceps delivery must be considered. The operator should evaluate the patient, her pelvis, and her labor pattern. He or she should also make an assessment of fetal status, including general condition, estimation of size, and determination of position, attitude, station, and degree of molding. Also important are the available facilities, services, and support staff. Finally, the operator's knowledge of the instruments, as well as his or her personal skill and limitations, should be weighed in the choices.

The initial choice is of the general course of action, namely, abdominal delivery, vaginal forceps delivery, trial of forceps, or vacuum extractor. Next, the choice of instrument must be made. Last, during performance of the procedure, choices of technique become necessary. The choice of delivery site must be made as well, depending on the availability of neonatal intensive care.

As previously stated, the elective and low forceps procedures have been shown to have results that are at least equivalent to those of spontaneous vaginal delivery. Midforceps procedures have fetal results comparable to those of cesarean delivery, particularly when the procedures are performed for similar indications. Although there is general agreement on the advantage of the "easy" midforceps delivery, a considerable problem exists in the prospective determination of which case should be "easy." With a problem case, collection and consideration of all the available clinical information should result in a greatly decreased incidence of the unanticipated difficult midforceps procedure that, in retrospect, should have been avoided. Certainly, if one is not reasonably certain, there is reason for cautious trial forceps (or a "trial of forceps").

The use of the term *failed forceps* is not advised. That specific negative term can stigmatize by implying that the procedure was abandoned after repeated attempts proved it to be impossible. Historically, *failed forceps* has suggested judgmental error, bad obstetrics, and possibly negligence. A *trial of forceps*, on the other hand, connotes a tentative attempt at a forceps delivery with the reservation to alter treatment if potentially dangerous resistance or difficulty is met. Performed with care and caution, usually with a double setup or as preparations are being made for cesarean delivery, it can prove fruitful and safe.

A forceps trial is not indicated for inlet dystocia or other problems at the inlet. Conditions such as a known pelvic abnormality with apparent fetopelvic disproportion, a brow presentation, a chin posterior face presentation, many previously diagnosed fetal anomalies, and a dead fetus with postmortem changes should not be considered for a trial of forceps, for obvious reasons. Indications for a trial of forceps should be critically considered in the case of labor arrests with the vertex at mid-pelvic level (ie, with a biparietal diameter at the plane of greatest pelvic dimensions and the hollow of the sacrum not filled). An appreciably higher incidence of depressed infants, shoulder dystocia, and maternal trauma can result in these instances. Protraction disorders treated by midforceps intervention are stated to be associated with an increased incidence of perinatal mortality. The procedure in such cases should be assessed with proper gravity.

In appropriate circumstances and with the availability of abdominal delivery in case of negative results, a trial of forceps is a valuable and eminently acceptable procedure. After evaluation of all available data, a gentle and judicious trial at low or midforceps level may be carried out. A careful attempt at application, rotation as necessary, and traction do not injure an infant. Injury is the result of force applied to tissues that resist that force, regardless of the reason. That resistance can be felt and is quite obvious. If the operator refuses to apply force of injurious quantity, injury cannot occur.

In the case of the premature and low-birth-weight infant, forceps were once believed to provide protection from trauma and its potential neurologic sequelae. Some recent studies have demonstrated cesarean delivery to be preferable when estimated fetal weight is in the very-low-birth-weight range (less than 1,500 g) or when the presentation is other than vertex. Estimation of fetal weight can become critical to proper management strategy, and ultrasound evaluation should be used, despite the possible (<10%) error rate. In the infant weighing more than 1,500 g, whether premature or small for gestational age, the advantage of cesarean delivery is not present. In this group of infants, no significant difference is reported between spontaneous and low forceps delivery, and decisions should be individualized for each case. It appears that fetal head compression is not a major determinant of intraventricular hemorrhage.

There is a growing body of evidence that, in most instances, modern delivery methods have little relationship to infant outcome. Considerably more important are other factors that may contribute to neonatal depression and the skill of perinatal management. Close collaboration between the obstetrician and the neonatologist is essential to improved results.

Choice of Instrument

Given a proper case for delivery with forceps, an operator must choose the kind of instrument most suitable for the conditions. Delivery may be accomplished with only one, or at most two, varieties of forceps. Other factors being equal, however, a greater degree of success should be obtained with a knowledge of the advantages and a discrimination in the use of the various kinds of forceps. Several kinds of forceps, both old and new, have peculiar advantages under certain conditions. The unique clinical advantages of each instrument are lost if one attempts to do everything with a single forceps.

In delivery with forceps under proper conditions, two features are of prime importance. First is the application of the forceps to the fetal head. Second, assuming that rotation of 45 degrees or less is required, is the traction used in accomplishing the delivery. These two acts determine the manipulation and effort required and, consequently, the associated trauma.

In a proper cephalic application, the blades should fit the head as accurately as possible. They should lie evenly against the sides of the head, reaching from the parietal bosses to, and beyond, the malar eminences, symmetrically covering the spaces between the orbits and the ears. There should be no extra pressure at any one point, so that pressure is evenly distributed and directed to the least vulnerable areas.

In the choice of an instrument with which a good application can be obtained, much depends on a correct diagnosis of the amount of molding; the position, station, and attitude of the head; and the type of pelvis. On molded heads, the best application is obtained with blades that have a long, tapering cephalic curve such that found in a Simpson-type forceps with parallel shanks. Those with a short, full curve, such as that found in an Elliot-type forceps with overlapping shanks, do not fit evenly, causing pressure points, and often they are not anchored below the malar eminences, consequently causing cutting or slipping. In considering the position of the head, the instrument to be chosen is the one that gives the correct application with the least effort. When the occiput is anterior, the application is, as a rule, easily made, and any blade that fulfills the requirements of the molding may be used. For other positions and presentations, there are special considerations with the various forceps operations. A head in the upper part of a flat pelvis or in a pelvis with a straight sacrum may be angulated in such a position that a cephalic application cannot be obtained.

Traction also plays a very important part in the choice of forceps. To use the least force, traction must be in the pelvic axis. This may be done manually, but it is best accomplished in all stations of the head with some form of axis traction forceps. Even in outlet forceps, axis traction is helpful in eliminating wasted force. To some, axis traction suggests a difficult operation with a complicated instrument. For this reason, it is often neglected in the average case, although the advantages are admitted. The classical forceps, without axis traction, are frequently used with the maximum force, aided by the Pajot or the Saxtorph maneuver. Axis traction forceps, however, tend to keep the force in the plane of least resistance, thereby diminishing the total effort required as well as the potential for injury.

In the selection of an instrument that fulfills the requirements of application and traction, there are many excellent forceps from which to choose. Some are simple, others complicated. All have one or more good points that justify their use when properly chosen. Some are so similar that there is very little choice between them. Various localities tend to have their favorites. Most modern forceps of the classical type generally follow one of two constructions: the shanks overlap and the blades have a short, cephalic curve, as in the Elliot; or the shanks are separated and the blades have a long, tapering curve, as in the Simpson. Not all of them, however, have axis traction. This disadvantage can be overcome in some by the use of the Bill axis traction handle.

For easy extractions from outlet or low level, the thin, solid blades of the Tucker-McLane (Elliot type) forceps are popular with some obstetricians. These instruments tend to fit best on small, rounder, less molded heads. They are easy to apply and remove but may slip owing to lack of anchorage below the malar eminences. On molded heads, they may exert pressure on two points: the zygoma and the parietal boss. The result may be a cut just in front of the ear or the later appearance of a localized parietal periostitis. The Luikart modification, with an indented fenestration on the inner surface of the solid blade, minimizes this disadvantage and is favored by many for elective forceps. On occasion, what is thought to be an easy outlet forceps later proves to be a molded head in which the biparietal diameter is at or above the ischial spines. The operator then wishes that a fenestrated blade had originally been chosen.

Most cases requiring delivery by forceps are in primiparous or multiparous women with a prolonged labor, and more molding should be anticipated. With increased molding of the head, the separated shanks and longer, tapered cephalic curve of the Simpson-type forceps make it the preferred instrument. The toes of the blades can seat well below the malar eminences, preventing pressure points and slipping.

In low and midforceps operations, more frequently than in outlet procedures, the position as well as the shape of the head must be considered in the choice of a suitable instrument. The rules for anterior positions are the same in all stations of the head, with emphasis on axis traction. With a fetal head in transverse arrest, some operators have developed skill in the use of manual rotation or the wandering maneuver with a classical instrument. It is not uncommon to find a head that cannot be rotated manually without displacement or one that refuses to remain anterior during the process of applying the second blade and locking the handles. In the wandering maneuver, the anterior blade occasionally hits the brow, causing the occiput to rotate backward. This may result in a brow-mastoid application, which no amount of manipulation will entirely correct. To simplify this procedure, a special type of forceps is available: the Kielland. The chief advantage of this instrument is the ease with which an accurate cephalic application can be obtained.

As previously noted (see Chapter 5, "Special Instruments"), several other instruments may be available that may supply the advantages of single application for attitude correction, rotation, and traction from transverse as well as posterior positions. In posterior positions, the single accurate application without displacement of the head, as well as semi-axis traction pull after rotation, with the Kielland forceps involve less manipulation than the Scanzoni maneuver or manual rotation. The upside-down, direct application of the Kielland forceps to an occiput posterior head permits rotation and extraction without readjustment of the blades. Exceptions to the procedure would be a marked anthropoid or android pelvis, in which case, because of limited space, it is considered necessary to deliver the posterior occiput as such, without anterior rotation. Here, a

Simpson-type instrument with axis traction is preferable to satisfy the requirements for molding and the need for an instrument with a good pelvic curve and better traction. If a Scanzoni maneuver is chosen, the solid-blade, Elliot-type instrument is preferred as a rotator in the first stage of the procedure.

Medical–Legal Aspects

In consideration of a legal problem and, in fact, of good medical practice, it is important to document forceps procedures. The indications for the procedure should be outlined to the patient and entered in the medical record. This discussion with the patient and/or relatives should be noted in the chart progress notes; it can simulate and indicate informed consent. The pertinent factors of predelivery and postdelivery fetal status, station, position, and attitude; the instrument and the type of forceps procedure; and the degree of difficulty should be recorded in a delivery note. The operator is also advised to make use of the laboratory facilities in unusual cases. Scalp pH readings in problem labors, cord pH at delivery, and pathologic examination of the placenta can offer potentially supporting evidence to the obstetrician, which is equally important as the monitor record.

The tendency is for the legal system to ascribe a damaged child to the procedure or its performance, rather than to the circumstances that indicated the procedure. The malpractice suit is settled by "the preponderance of evidence." The operator must attempt to prove that the damage was incurred either before or after the procedure in question. This is obviously not easy, particularly in the emotionally charged situation of a defective child.

To paraphrase Dr. M. Rosen: Do good or bad obstetrics and get a good result, and you don't get sued. Do good or bad obstetrics and get a bad result, and you do get sued; so you might as well do good obstetrics.

Conclusion

The obstetrician is currently confronted by increasing demands from outside as well as within the profession, causing the specialty to be even more demanding than in the past. Forceps delivery, previously considered the hallmark of the obstetrician, is a valuable and necessary skill that should be taught and made available as a management strategy alternative for all deliveries. The decrease in forceps learning experiences, whether due to the decrees of program directors or to pressure from consumers, results in inexperienced operators whose only safe option in a difficult situation is abdominal delivery. This raises maternal cost, risks, and sequelae without improvement of fetal results.

Outlet and low forceps procedures, including elective forceps, have been demonstrated to have results at least as good as those obtained with spontaneous delivery. The same is true of midforceps contrasted to cesarean delivery. Thus, the object of forceps delivery does not connote a "trade-off" of fetal versus maternal injury.

Observation of the prerequisites for forceps delivery is mandatory. The more obvious ruptured membranes, engaged head, fully dilated and retracted cervix, and appropriate anesthesia, equipment, and support personnel need no further comment. A working knowledge of obstetric pelvic architecture is necessary to predict labor events and plan management. The initial pelvic examination during labor should include a clinical pelvimetry, checking the information gained during the patient's prenatal course. A recheck of the pelvis after delivery, particularly with conduction anesthesia, is excellent for self-instruction. This can also be done from the opposite direction during cesarean delivery.

Because accurate application is so extremely important to safe forceps control of the fetal head, the intrapartum observations of position, attitude, and station assume greater import. If landmarks are obscured, the direction of the sagittal suture can at least be identified (eg, sagittal suture in left oblique, running from right anterior to left posterior quadrant). This information can be significant to the later course of labor, as can the observation of the fetal attitude of flexion or extension. The diagnosis of asynclitism and of the level of the biparietal diameter, as well as evaluation of labor for abnormalities of dilatation or descent, are equally significant prerequisites to forceps use. These factors should be looked for and recorded.

Applying proper traction while minimizing compression is essential. Rotation to occiput anterior is usual and is accomplished by manual, instrumental, or a combination method before traction. Traction must be made in the axis of the pelvis to minimize the force required and the potential for injury. The direction of traction is critical and is properly applied perpendicular to the plane of the pelvis at the level of the biparietal diameter Traction force must be controlled and carefully applied, because force is required for injury and the objective is an atraumatic delivery.

Certainly not the least of the prerequisites for forceps delivery is the operator's knowledge of the instruments and choice of forceps to fit the individual case. Most experienced operators have had cases in which delivery was too difficult with one instrument but was completed successfully with another. It rarely takes more than one such experience to convince one that there is indeed a choice of forceps to suit the case.

Any intelligent operator with ordinary obstetric skills can perform outlet, low, and even midforceps procedures. With observance of the prerequisites and a cautious, gentle approach, most procedures are almost surprisingly simple when properly performed. The operator must think in a few terms with which he or she may be unfamiliar. First of these is biparietal diameter: the measurement of the head that must be moved through the pelvis. The biparietal diameter contains the pivot point of the head and is on the long axis of the head. Second is the axis of the pelvis, to which traction should be perpendicular, and the long axis of the head, to which traction should be parallel. Third is the toes of the forceps blade rather than the handles, because the toes must remain as close as possible to the center of the pelvis. The last consideration is the plane of least resistance with application, rotation, and traction.

The operator must be prepared to abandon an unusually difficult procedure, evaluating the reasons for the difficulty, trying a different approach, and even allowing further labor or moving to abdominal delivery. The use of increased force is not an acceptable alternative. It is difficult to cause injury if one takes the force out of forceps.

After all forceps deliveries, it is advisable to examine the infant for marks or signs of trauma. With most procedures, little if any marking should be visible. When marks are visible, the symmetry and location should reassure the operator as to the correctness of application and traction. Variations from optimal technique will often be visible for several hours and can serve as a valuable learning tool. For example, if the forceps are not directed far enough below the horizontal in an oblique or transverse position, extra pressure on the anterior cheek will have marked that cheek.

Concerning the medical–legal problem, the physician is advised to explain and document all circumstances of the forceps delivery. An estimate of the degree of difficulty of the procedure should be recorded. As much laboratory support as possible should be used. In view of the currently prevailing patient prejudice concerning obstetric forceps, patient education is indicated, certainly postpartum, if not antepartum or intrapartum. In this respect, an innocent history question, "Was your delivery normal or by forceps?", can be prejudicial and potentially dangerous.

Studies related to forceps have been confusing and notoriously difficult to compare in the past. Opposite conclusions have been reported from presumably similar procedures performed by different investigators. At least part of the confusion has been due to a previously inadequate classification, a situation that should now be corrected. We are certain that forceps deliveries will continue to occupy a major place in the practice of obstetrics, important in the armamentarium lucinae.

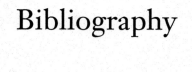

Bibliography

American College of Obstetricians and Gynecologists. Delivery by vacuum extraction. ACOG Committee Opinion 208. Washington, DC: ACOG, 1998

American College of Obstetricians and Gynecologists. Operative vaginal delivery. ACOG Practice Bulletin 17. Washington, DC: ACOG, 2000

Benedetti TJ. Birth injury and method of delivery. N Engl J Med 1999; 341:1758–1759

Bofill JA, Rust OA, Perry KG, Roberts WE, Martin RW, Morrison JC. Operative vaginal delivery: a survey of fellows of ACOG. Obstet Gynecol 1996;88:1007–1010

Bofill JA, Rust OA, Schorr SJ, Brown RC, Roberts WE, Morrison JC. A randomized trial of two vacuum extraction techniques. Obstet Gynecol 1997;89:758–762

Carmona F, Martinez-Roman S, Manau D, Cararach V, Iglesias X. Immediate maternal and neonatal effects of low-forceps delivery according to the new criteria of the American College of Obstetricians and Gynecologists compared with spontaneous vaginal delivery in term pregnancies. Am J Obstet Gynecol 1995;173:55–59

Chan CC, Malathi I, Yeo GS. Is the vacuum extractor really the instrument of first choice? Aust N Z J Obstet Gynaecol 1999;39:305–309

Eustace DL. James Young Simpson: the controversy surrounding the presentation of his Air Tractor (1848-1849). J R Soc Med 1993;86:660–663

Feldman DM, Borgida AF, Sauer F, Rodis JF. Rotational versus nonrotational forceps: maternal and neonatal outcomes. Am J Obstet Gynecol 1999;181:1185–1187

Florentino-Pineda I, Ezhuthachan SG, Sineni LG, Kumar SP. Subgaleal hemorrhage in the newborn infant associated with silicone elastomer vacuum extractor. J Perinatol 1994;14:95–100

Hankins GD, Rowe TF. Operative vaginal delivery—year 2000. Am J Obstet Gynecol 1996;175:275–282

Hankins GD, Leicht T, Van Hook J, Uckan EM. The role of forceps rotation in maternal and neonatal injury. Am J Obstet Gynecol 1999; 180:231–234

Johanson RB, Heycock E, Carter J, Sultan AH, Walklate K, Jones PW. Maternal and child health after assisted vaginal delivery: five-year follow up of a randomised controlled study comparing forceps and ventouse. Br J Obstet Gynaecol 1999;106:544–549

Kuit JA, Eppinga HG, Wallenburg HC, Huikeshoven FJ. A randomized comparison of vacuum extraction delivery with a rigid and a pliable cup. Obstet Gynecol 1993;82:280–284

Peleg D, Kennedy CM, Merrill D, Zlatnik FJ. Risk of repetition of a severe perineal laceration. Obstet Gynecol 1999;93:1021–1024

Robertson PA, Laros RK Jr, Zhao RL. Neonatal and maternal outcome in low-pelvic and midpelvic operative deliveries. Am J Obstet Gynecol 1990;162:1436–1442; discussion 1442–1444

Robson S, Pridmore B. Have Kielland forceps reached their "use by" date? Aust N Z J Obstet Gynaecol 1999;39:301–304

Royal College of Obstetricians and Gynaecologists. Instrumental vaginal delivery. RCOG Guideline 26. London: RCOG, 2000

Teng FY, Sayre JW. Vacuum extraction: does duration predict scalp injury? Obstet Gynecol 1997;89:281–285

Towner D, Castro MA, Eby-Wilkens E, Gilbert WM. Effect of mode of delivery in nulliparous women on neonatal intracranial injury. N Engl J Med 1999;341:1709–1714

Trends in cesarean section, forceps deliveries and vacuum extraction in the United States, 1970-1998. Unpublished chart compiled by ACOG Resource Center from National Center for Health Statistics data, 2000

Vintzileos AM, Nochimson DJ, Antsaklis A, Varvarigos I, Guzman ER, Knuppel RA. Effect of vacuum extraction on umbilical cord blood acid-base measurements. J Matern Fetal Med 1996;5:11–17

Wesley BD, van den Berg BJ, Reece EA. The effect of forceps delivery on cognitive development. Am J Obstet Gynecol 1993;169:1091–1095

Williams MC, Knuppel RA, O'Brien WF, Weiss A, Spellacy WN, Pietrantoni M. Obstetric correlates of neonatal retinal hemorrhage. Obstet Gynecol 1993;81:688–694

Yancey MK, Herpolsheimer A, Jordan GD, Benson WL, Brady K. Maternal and neonatal effects of outlet forceps delivery compared with spontaneous vaginal delivery in term pregnancies. Obstet Gynecol 1991;78:646–650

Index

Note: Page numbers followed by *f*, *n*, and *t* indicate figures, notes, and tables, respectively.